Healing Herbs
for
Arthritis and Rheumatism

by
Alexandra Donson

  FFORBEZ PUBLICATIONS   VANCOUVER, CANADA

STERLING PUBLISHING CO., INC.   NEW YORK

First published in Canada in 1982 by Fforbez Publications Ltd., 2133 Quebec Street, Vancouver, B.C. V5T 2Z9

First published in the United States of America in 1982 by Sterling Publishing Co., Inc., Two Park Avenue, New York, N.Y. 10016

© 1982 by Alexandra Donson
Printed in Canada

Typesetting by Bev Ruhl
Cover Design by Chris Hanlon
Art by Alexandra Donson

Canadian Cataloguing in Publication Data

Donson, Alexandra.
Healing herbs for arthritis and rheumatism

Includes index.
Bibliography: p.
Fforbez ISBN 0-88976-062-4
Sterling ISBN 0-8069-7578-4

1. Arthritis. 2. Rheumatism. 3. Herbs - Therapeutic use. I. Title.
RC933.A2D65   616.7'2   C81-091098-5

This book is dedicated to
Dr. David T. Suzuki, geneticist,
because he is so great
and to our parents who love us.

Tibetan Prayer to Forgiveness

Spiritual son of Buddhas, Padma Sambhava,
   O victorious one,
Forgive me for handing on your instruction
Which is like purified gold
To others, for the sake of the sick and the
   teaching.
Bless this faithful dKon-mchhog rGyal-mt'san
To become a most excellent benefactor of beings.

Contents

PART THREE: ORIENTAL ORIGINS OF HERBAL HEALING

Acknowledgements

I am very grateful for all the help I have received in writing this volume. In all the years I have been studying plants, many times in the company of other collectors, moments have not been wasted to constantly say prayers for those I love. This work has been gathered together as a result.

I would particularly like to thank the following individuals:

Mr. Richard Copley, Asst. Professor of Geography at the University of British Columbia, who taught me to understand many of the ways of the Japanese culture.

Abraham Apukark Anghik Ruben, Canadian Eskimo artist, who taught me to understand the spiritual values of nature.

David Piqtoukun Ruben, his brother.

Mary Vorvis, for her quick, efficient work in typing the final manuscript.

Nicholas Bergen, for his metaphysical advice on matters of consequence.

Lianne Chu, artist with cloth, who helped me with the first original volume of this work.

David B. Roberts, woodcarver; may he always shine with his quiet spirit.

University of British Columbia Librarians, for all their wonderful assistance.

Ken Mah, for financial support.

Gordon Soules, publisher, for all his encouragement and help in the publishing world.

Mr. Ching Lieu, Tai Chi Master, for teaching me greatly about the nature of herbs.

Gretchen Perk, school teacher, whose enthusiasm for this Holistic Herbal Healing Age gives me a great deal of laughter.

Ted Pappas, for his constant moral and financial support which made the first draft of this book possible.

Mrs. Virginia Black, secretary of University Hill United Church, my dear friend, whose constant patience, guidance and prayers for me and my efforts guided me to the completion of this work.

The Tibetan Archives in Dharmasala, India, for their promptness in sending material.

Mr. Don Sui, of the Universal Buddhist Temple, who amazes me with his knowledge of healing.

Honorable Professor W.S. Fung, President of the Universal Buddhist Temple, and Honorable Mr. Lu, for their blessings and patience with my incessant demands, and their knowledge of plants and healing.

Leon Zolbrod, Professor of Asian Studies at the University of British Columbia, for his translation of poetry into Japanese and his wonderful knowledge of Japanese literature.

John Tanner, astronomer, for his celestial companionship in the field.

Kumar and Owl Clearmorning, little children mountaineers, to whom I dedicate my love.

Dean Mah, traveller, who reminds me that we are still children.

Costa Pappas, for his constant affection and devotion in matters of herbal use.

Isaac Asimov, our hero, for his astronomical versatility and inspiration.

Ronald N. Labonte, Kurtis Venel and Carolyn Griffiths, for their assistance with proofreading the manuscript.

Peter Zebroff, my wonderful publisher, for giving so much to me and doing so much for me.

Jim Wright, for all his courage, strength, wonderful support, endless help and co-operation in seeing this work through.

Beth Tetzel, my editor, for her graceful, untiring patience and enthusiasm with the proofreading and all those things that are very important in publishing a book.

Quick Herbal Reference

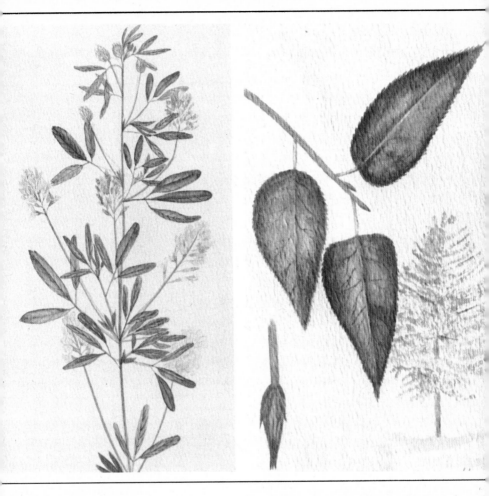

Alfalfa
(Medicago sativa)
Cleanses the body of
arthritis. (See page 37.)

Balm of Gilead
(Populus balsamifera)
Prevents rheumatism. (See
page 42.)

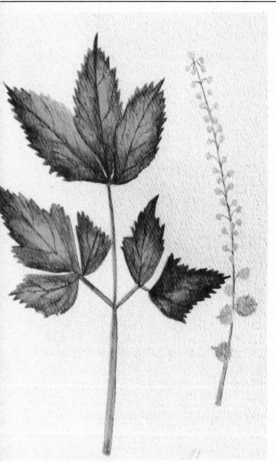
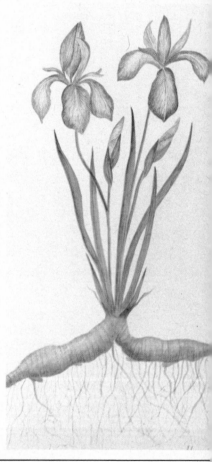

Black Cohosh
(Cimicifuga racemosa)
A tonic and liver
stimulant; good for
rheumatic pain. (See page
44.)

Blue Flag
(Iris versicolor)
Used for advanced
rheumatism and feeble
condition. (See page 46.)

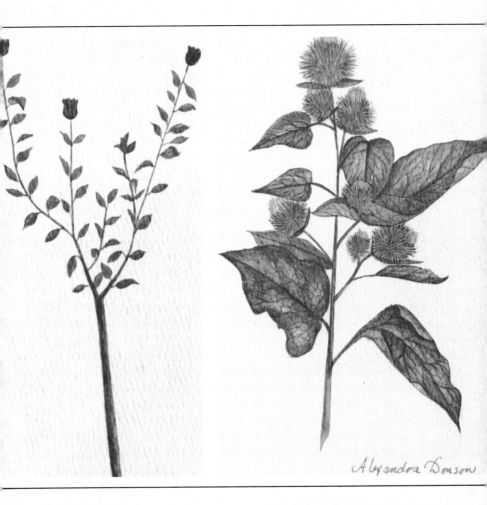

Alexandra Dowson

Buchu
(Barosma betulina)
For advanced rheumatism; a blood purifier. (See page 48.)

Burdock Root
(Arctium lappa)
Improves health, removes pain in joints. It is used in cooking and as a poultice. (See page 49.)

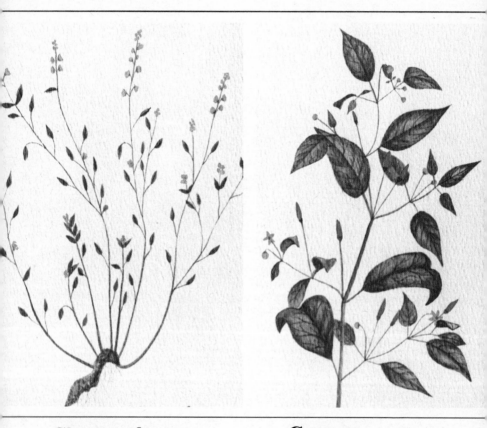

Chaparral
(Larrea tridentata)
A cell restorative; cleans blood and restores digestive organs to proper functioning. (See page 54.)

Cayenne
(Capsicum minimum)
Used for quick relief of arthritic pain, both as a liniment and internally. Improves the heart. (See page 52.)

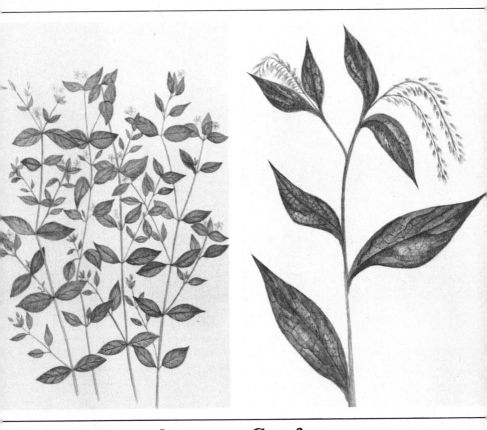

Chickweed
(Stellaria media)
A body cleanser; relieves arthritis. (See page 56.)

Comfrey
(Symphytum officinale)
A rapid cell healer; relieves arthritis. (See page 59.)

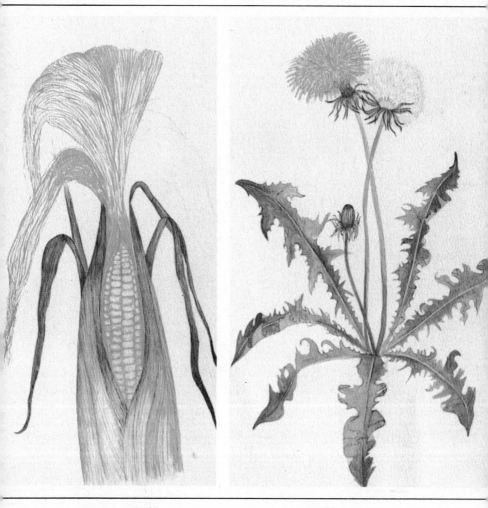

Corn Silk
(Stigmata maydis)
Quickly eliminates uric acid. Used for all forms of arthritis. (See page 62.)

Dandelion
(Taraxacum officinale)
Quickly eliminates uric acid. (See page 64.)

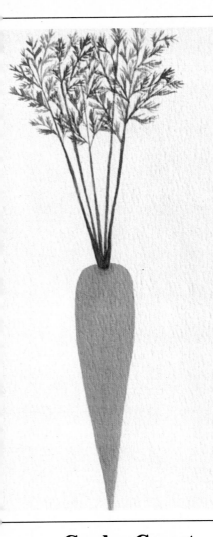

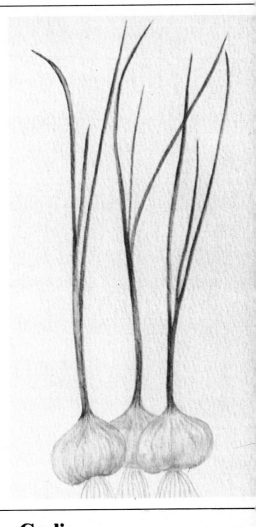

Garden Carrot
(Oxheart chanteney nantes)
Cleans blood. (See page 67.)

Garlic
(Allium sativum)
Cleans blood, improves digestion. (See page 68.)

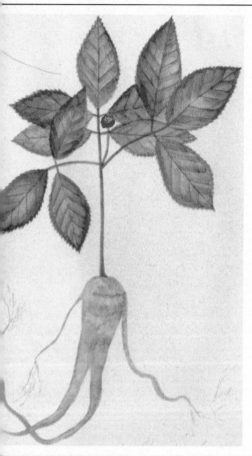 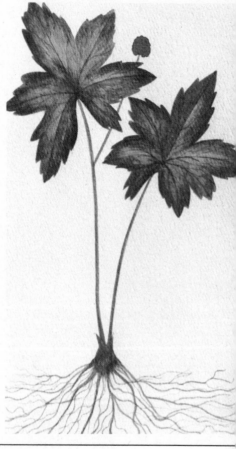

Ginseng
(Panax quinquefolium)
A tonic; improves health and promotes longevity. (See page 70.)

Golden Seal
(Hydrastis canadensis)
Used to relieve inflammation and pain. (See page 73.)

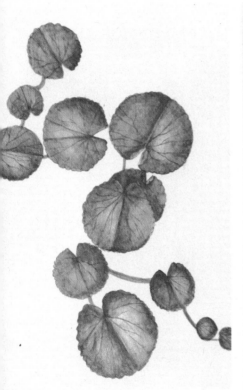 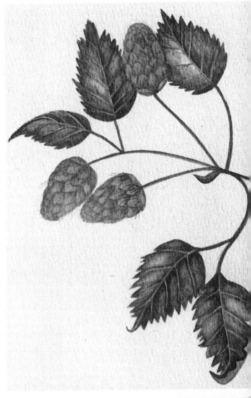

Gotu Kola
(Centella asiatica)
Good for the brain and nervous system; promotes longevity. Eliminates rheumatism. (See page 76.)

Hops
(Humulus lupulus)
Beer as tonic; improves bladder and kidney functions. Used to heal rheumatism and inflammations. (See page 78.)

17

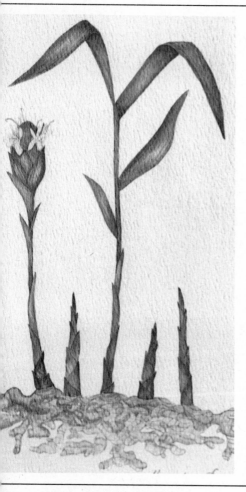

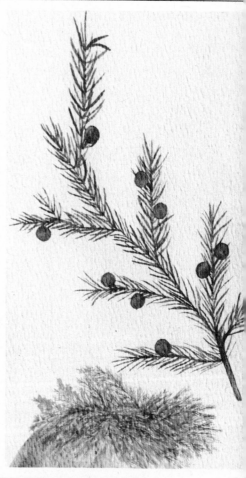

Jamaica Ginger
(Zingiber officinale)
Rheumatism preventative;
tonic. (See page 80.)

Juniper Berry
(Juniperis communis)
Rheumatism preventative;
tonic. (See page 81.)

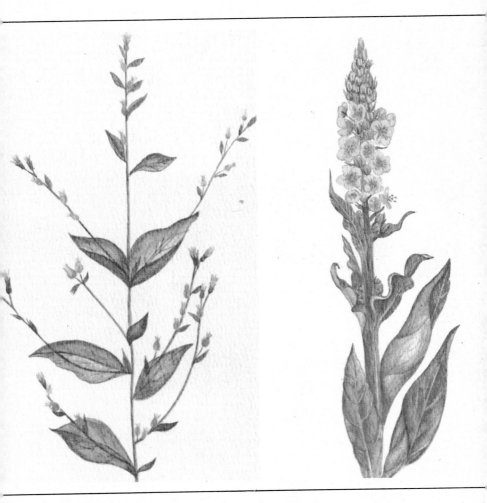

Lobelia
(Lobelia inflata)
Tranquilizer; pain killer for rheumatism. (See page 83.)

Mullein
(Verbascum thapsus)
Tranquilizer, muscle relaxant; removes rheumatic pain. (See page 85.)

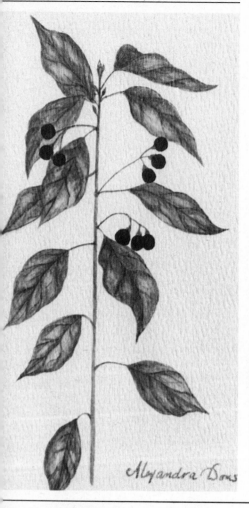

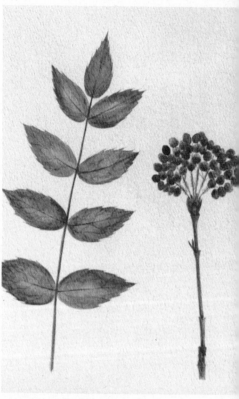

Myrrh
(Commiphora myrrha)
A stimulant and disinfectant, myrrh has a warming effect and can be used as a liniment. (See page 87.)

Oregon Grape
(Berberis aquifolium)
Eliminates rheumatism. (See page 89.)

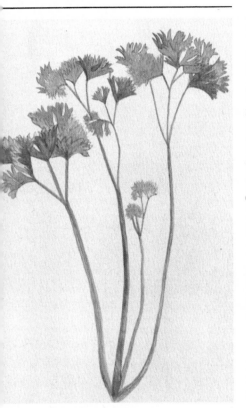

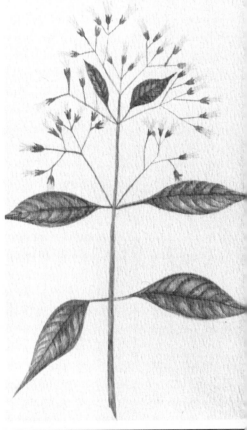

Parsley
(Carum petroselinum)
A blood cleanser; relieves arthritis. (See page 90.)

Peruvian Bark
(Cinchona calisaya)
Removes pain in acute rheumatism. (See page 92.)

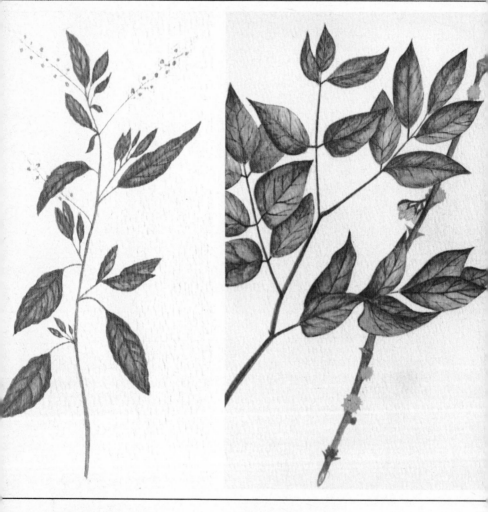

Poke Root
(Phytolaca decandra)
A tonic for chronic, advanced rheumatism. (See page 94.)

Prickly Ash
(Zanthoxylum americanum)
A mild tranquilizer; strengthens the heart and nervous system. Used for chronic and rheumatoid arthritis. (See page 96.)

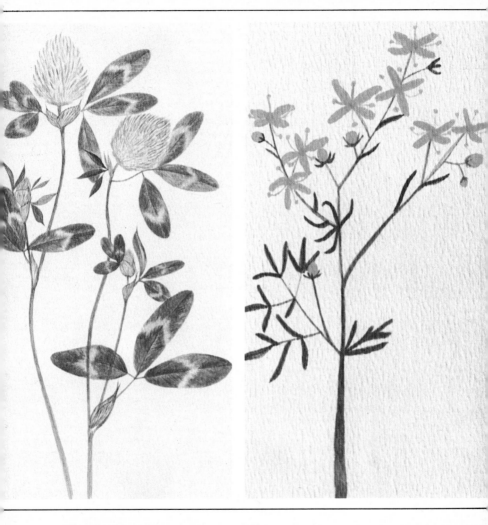

Red Clover
(Trifolium pratense)
A rapid blood cleaner; removes uric acid. (See page 98.)

Rue
(Ruta graveolins)
Used to heal painful external joints. (See page 100.)

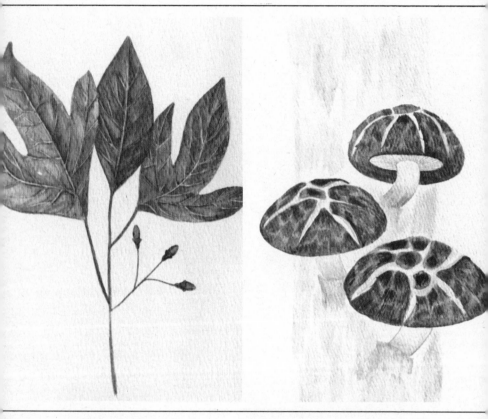

Sassafras
(Sassafras officinale)
A blood purifier, body cleanser and tonic. (See page 102.)

Shiitake Mushrooms
(Lentinus edodes)
Relieves rheumatism and cleans the body. (See page 104.)

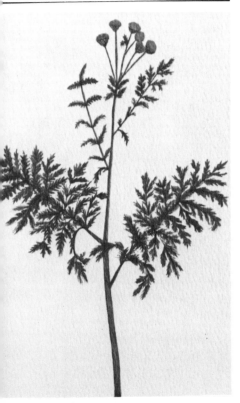

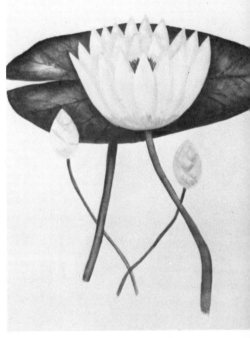

Tansy
(Tanacetum vulgare)
A tonic and relaxant, tansy can also be used as a poultice. (See page 106.)

White Pond Lily
(Nymphaea alba)
A body, bladder and kidney cleanser, the white pond lily is also an excellent tonic. (See page 108.)

25

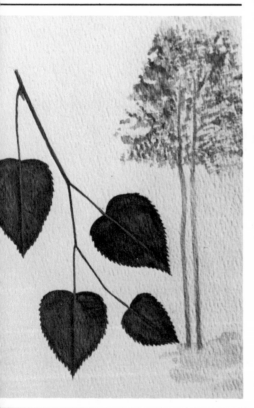

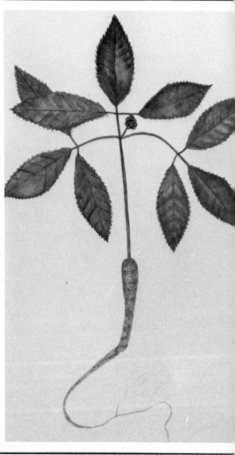

White Poplar
(Populus tremuloides)
Good for swellings and acute rheumatism. (See page 111.)

Wild Ginseng
(Aralia nudicaulis)
Promotes longevity. Can be used in any arthritis or rheumatism healing program. (See page 113.)

PART ONE:
HERBAL HEALING

Taittariya Upanishad III, 10

Bravo! Bravo! Bravo!
I am food! I am food! I am food!
I am an eater of food! I am an eater of food! I am
an eater of food!
I am a maker of verses! I am a maker of verses! I
am a maker of verses!
I am first-born of the universal order,
Earlier than the gods, in the navel of immortality!
Whoso gives me away, he, verily, has succoured
me.
I who am food eat the eater of good!
I have overcome the whole world!

He who knows this shines with a golden light.

*Hindu Scriptures, p. 144. (Toronto, Ontario: J.M. Dent and Sons
(Canada) Ltd.) Reprinted by permission of the publishers.*

Introduction

Although modern medical chemicals help to cure many diseases, they do not possess the same healing qualities as herbal prescriptions. A single molecule pulled out of a plant or manufactured in a laboratory does not have the same healing properties as the plant itself. In some cases, another vitamin or enzyme in the plant is essential to trigger its action. A plant, berry or piece of bark may contain up to twenty ingredients which interact to produce a healing effect. The small size of the molecules in many plants allows them to be easily absorbed and eliminated by the body.

Most modern drugs consist of one or more isolated molecules surrounded by a sugar base. This type of medicine forces the body to expend greater energy to utilize the chemical because it is not aided by the plant's other natural ingredients. Artificially manufactured drugs can be especially harsh on the kidneys. Although these drugs provide relief from symptoms, they can be extremely difficult to digest. The chemical toxins left in the body after absorption are even harder to eliminate.

When deciding whether or not to take a drug, consider both its curative power and safety. What side effects will it have on your body? Will it promote your body's overall health while healing is taking place?

In most instances, it takes longer to remove a disease using herbal methods than it does using modern drugs. But herbal healing has few side effects or complications, has longer-lasting benefits and usually leaves the body in a healthier state.

Herbalists have never claimed that any one herb cures any one disease. What herbs do is to stimulate the resistance of the body's own tissue to the disease or condition.

Causes of Joint Disorders

Some joint disorders are caused by the incomplete breakdown of chemicals in the body and the body's inability to eliminate this waste matter in its unchanged state. The incomplete breakdown of toxic matter forms uric acid, excess mucus and toxic waste. This interferes with proper digestion.

A poor diet—one which relies heavily on refined foods, starch and animal protein—causes the urea to be left incompletely transformed. These foods are acid-producing and must be balanced by a neutralizer (such as sodium) or an alkaline substance.

Calcium is the element most frequently associated with joint trouble. When calcium has not been dissolved in the blood, it settles, undissolved, in the joints, especially the hands and feet. Excess calcium in the blood is caused by an acid/alkaline imbalance. This means that other chemicals must be added to restore the blood's balance. Constant circulation of sodium over the hard calcium deposits will eventually remove them.

Types of Joint Disorders

Acute arthritis: An attack of redness, swelling, pain and heat. It may appear in any joint.

Allergic arthritis: A sudden reaction in the joints caused by an allergy. This reaction may be caused by eating certain foods or taking certain medicines.

Arthritis: Joint inflammation.

Bursitis: Inflammation of a bursa, especially one located between a bony prominence and a muscle or tendon (commonly occurs in the shoulder, but can occur elsewhere, such as in the knee, arm or hand).

Chronic arthritis or rheumatism: Arthritis or rheumatism which has lasted for many months or years. This includes chronic swellings or stiffness.

Degenerative arthritis: Generally a problem of the elderly. A chronic, usually progressive, joint disease involving multiple joints, characterized by the destruction of joint cartilage and other degenerative changes.

Gonorrheal arthritis: Inflammation of the joints resulting from a severe case of gonorrhea.

Gout: Paroxysmal metabolic disease marked by acute arthritis and inflammation of the joints.

Hemophilic arthritis: Inflammation and stiffness caused by chronic bleeding into a joint.

Lumbago: A general term for dull, aching pain across the loins.

Menopausal arthritis: Inflammation in the joints of women during menopause.

Muscular rheumatism: Pain or stiffness of the muscles.

Neuralgia: Pain along the route of a nerve.

Neuritis: One or more inflamed nerve trunks.

Osteoarthritis: A chronic disease that causes bone and cartilage degeneration and eventually produces deformation and impaired function.

Rheumatism: Soreness and stiffness of muscles and pain in joints and associated structures (a general term that is applied to both acute and chronic joint/muscle conditions).

Rheumatoid arthritis: A very common form of arthritis in which many of the joints are swollen simultaneously.

Sciatica: Pain along the sciatic nerve from the back of the thigh running down the inside of the leg.

Healing your Body

Herbs, like nature, work very slowly. They are extremely mild and are excellent for chronic conditions. The side effects of the herbs described in this book are negligible or nonexistent, especially those with a vegetable base, such as comfrey or alfalfa.

After your type of arthritis has been diagnosed, decide on a specific healing regimen. Since many herbs can be useful in removing any one disorder, select a tea which contains those herbs most effective in relieving your ailment. (See Part 2 for the tea recipes and a description of the healing properties of each herb. The Quick Herbal Reference and the Index will help you to find any specific information you desire.)

Once you have chosen a herb or herbal combination, try it for a minimum of three weeks, drinking one to two cups of tea or elixir per day. At this point the pain associated with arthritis should disappear. If you drink the tea regularly for three or four months, other improvements in your condition will become apparent. With a positive change in diet, using body-building elixirs and herbs, some forms of arthritis can be eliminated in one to two years.

Gathering Herbs

Plants for medicine should ideally be gathered in their original environment, the garden or forest. The natural nutrients provided by humus and the gardening provided by insects cannot be imitated in a chemically fertilized garden. Overly domesticated plants do not contain the same chemical components as their natural counterparts and may not have medicinal value.

Many wild herbs cannot easily be cultivated in a home garden. Plants get their mineral properties from the soil, so if you must grow your own herbs, gather soil from a forest, if possible, and use only organic compost. A number of the herbs listed in Part 2 can be grown in the home garden or even indoors.

When you should gather herbs depends on what part of the plant you want. Roots should be gathered in the late fall or early spring. This is the time when all of the plant's potency is stored in the root. Once growth starts, the root's energy is transferred to and shared with the leaves. Take care not to break the skin of the root so that the essential liquids and saps will remain in the plant.

The bark of trees and shrubs should be gathered in the late spring and summer, when the lifeblood of the plant is flowing through the cell walls.

The leaves of plants should be gathered before they begin to flower. This usually gives a sweeter tasting herb, and the energy has not yet been absorbed by the fruit. Leaves should be gathered whole. Be careful not to break the delicate vein structure or tear the stem away.

Flowers should be gathered in full bloom and, if odorous, while the fragrance still lingers.

Preserving Herbs

Carefully separate the roots and hang them up to dry in a warm, dark place. The drying time depends on the size of the root.

The strips of bark taken from trees should also be tied with string and hung in a warm, dark place.

Dry leaves quickly in order to conserve their properties. Place them on large cookie trays in a low-temperature oven for 12-15 hours, or tie them in bundles and hang them in a warm, dark place. After the leaves have dried, be careful not to break them. Put the whole leaves into a large airtight jar. Once broken up into tea, the leaves will stay fresh for several months in an airtight jar.

Preparing Green Drinks

The following drink is very refreshing and retains all the vitamins, minerals, enzymes and chlorophyl released from the leaves.

Green Outdoor Elixir

Take 2-3 handfuls of fresh green herbs and rinse them carefully. Pick off any leaves that are brown, retaining the fresh green ones.

Chop the leaves very finely to expose as much of the leaf vein as possible. Then put them into a bowl and mash them with a wooden spoon.

Put the mashed leaves into a gallon of water, cover and place in the hot sun. Let this mixture sit in the sun for 4-6 hours. Shake occasionally. Strain.

Drink in the sunshine. Ice cubes, honey and lemon juice may be added if desired.

Blender Drinks

Freshly gathered plants can also be put into a blender for a few seconds. Allow the liquid to stand for an hour or so before straining out the leaf pulp. Honey or soya sauce may be added for additional flavour.

Preparing Herb Teas

Herb teas should be prepared in either a porcelain or glass pot. *Never* use aluminum.

Bring water to a boil, then sprinkle the dried or fresh herb on top of the water. Cover the pot and remove it from the heat. Allow the tea to sit for 20 to 60 minutes before straining it into a teapot and serving it. Honey or soya sauce can be added for additional flavour.

Notes on Dosage

Herb amounts may be adjusted to suit the needs and stature of the indivudual. A small person will need less than will a very large individual. It is best to start with a low dosage and gradually build up to the required dose over a period of one to two weeks, especially with fresh juices, which are very potent. This gives the body time to adjust to the healing regime without causing it distress from too rapid a change in diet or too rapid a healing process.

If you forget to use herbs for a day or two, there will usually be enough medicine in your system to compensate for the omission. If, however, you skip one to two weeks while healing is required the original condition may reappear. Once you begin to take the herbs again healing will resume immediately.

Although capsules are more convenient than making tea, the tea has been found to be more easily and readily absorbed into the system.

Do not expect commercial bottled products to work in the same way as fresh herbs. Obtain fresh dried herbs from a herb shop or gather them yourself.

Herbal Fasting

The quickest method of cleaning and healing the body of rheumatism and other disorders is moderate fasting. Extreme fasting—drinking only water—can draw too many toxins into the eliminative system all at once, causing additional discomfort.

Moderate fasting deprives the body of protein and carbohydrates. This releases the body's energy to digest and eliminate waste tissue and accompanying toxic matter. It also allows the body to rest its overworked system and recuperate its strength with healing herbs. Since the body in a cleaned state is more receptive to the changes caused by healing herbs, regular fasting should be a part of any healing program.

Because the human body is self-rejuvenating and self-rebuilding, some disorders can be totally eliminated through fasting. It may take up to several years depending on the program you choose, but nature always comes through.

The body is constantly in a state of change; the food you eat today determines how healthy you will be in the following weeks and even years. Moderate fasting allows you to slowly eliminate the old and unhealthy cells in your body and replace them with new cells. This, in turn, helps you to live longer and enjoy good health. By making you sit up and take notice of the world around you, fasting also leads to greater spiritual awareness and joy.

It takes a long time for the diseased tissue to be dissolved and reabsorbed into the bloodstream for removal from the body, but eventually new tissue will replace the old. During this healing process the pain and problems of the disease will manifest themselves temporarily, but this will not last long and the reward is excellent health.

Before you undertake a fast, even if it will only last one or two days, improve your diet by eliminating animal protein, heavy starches and excessive stimulants such as coffee and tea. Fasting causes the rapid removal of fat with all its stored poisons. The body can only eliminate so many toxins and poisons at once, so acknowledge this limitation and don't give your body too much work to do too quickly.

During even moderate fasting some of the following symptoms usually appear: extreme elation, a sense of weakness, periodic irritability, coated tongue, nausea, bad breath, minor stomach aches, boils, or a slight rash. Drugs stored in your body (aspirin, penicillin, codeine, marijuana, etc.) will be released and you will re-experience their effects. Most of these symptoms are of short duration and need not cause concern. This is nature's way of telling you that your illness is on its way out of your body.

Rest often during a fast, as your body is working hard to help itself and should be given every chance to do so. If you fast for as long as a week, rest at least one or two hours every afternoon.

Fasting with Herbal Elixirs

If you drink elixirs during your fast, the nutrient level in your body will be high enough that you can carry on moderate activity without difficulty. Drink at least two quarts of liquid (elixirs and water) each day. Even very sick people can fast without losing strength if they drink elixirs because this removes the disorder and at the same time builds the blood and renews the cells.

Fasting has other positive effects. It neutralizes acids in the body and balances the acid/alkaline content of the blood. One begins to sleep very well at this point. High blood pressure drops immediately and usually becomes normal after one or two days of fasting. Digestion of food also becomes easier after a brief fast.

When you fast, do so with happiness. If you choose to fast for several days, try to spend the time in a beautiful, restful environment where you can relax and be happy.

End your fast very slowly, eating small meals of fresh salads and clear soups for at least two days. Breaking a fast too suddenly will wreak havoc with your digestive tract and undo the good of the fast.

The following recipes are for use during fasting.

Rheumatism Tea—Elixir for Mountain People

240 grams (8 oz.) Mu tea
480 grams (16 oz.) gypsum pound
60 grams (2 oz.) licorice
30 grams (1 oz.) dried ginseng powder (red)

30 grams (1 oz.) ginger
15 grams (½ oz.) burdock root

Boil all herbs except gypsum pound for 30 minutes; then add gypsum.

Green Buddha Rheumatism Tea

This tea strengthens blood circulation and the digestive system.

1 part cinnamon
1 part red ginseng powder
1 part Chinese red date
1 part ginger
1 part peony root
1 part licorice root
1 part burdock root

Put all the ingredients into a large pot of water. Bring to a boil and let steep for 30 minutes to an hour.

Soup for Buddha

2 L (8 cups) boiling water
30 ml (2 tbsp.) soya sauce
Green onions or garlic greens chopped finely
30 ml (2 tbsp.) powdered ginseng root (red)
10 ml (2 tsp.) sesame oil

Put all ingredients into a large bowl and pour boiling water over them. Let sit for five minutes and savour for one-half hour.

Soup of Heaven

2 L (8 cups) boiling water
Garlic or green onion greens chopped finely
8 large shiitake mushrooms
5 ml (1 tsp.) sesame oil
30 ml (2 tbsp.) soya sauce
10 ml (2 tsp.) Nori seaweed

Boil water and mushrooms for an hour. Remove mushrooms. Put in oil and soya sauce. Cook for 3 minutes. Pour into bowls and add greens. Sprinkle top with seaweed. Savour for one-half hour. Delicious.

PART TWO:
SPECIFIC HERBS
AND RECIPES

A university student, while visiting Gasan, asked him; "Have you ever read the Christian Bible?"

"No, read it to me," said Gasan.

The student opened the Bible and read from St. Matthew: "And why take ye thought for raiment? Consider the lilies of the field, how they grow. They toil not, neither do they spin, and yet I say unto you that even Solomon in all his glory was not arrayed like one of these. . . . Take therefore no thought for the morrow, for the morrow shall take thought for the things of itself."

Gasan said, "Whoever uttered those words I consider an enlightened man."

The student continued reading: "Ask and it shall be given you, seek and ye shall find, knock and it shall be opened unto you. For everyone that asketh receiveth and he that seeketh findeth, and to him that knocketh it shall be opened."

Gasan remarked, "That is excellent. Whoever said that is not far from Buddhahood."

Zen Flesh, Zen Bones by Paul Reps, p. 20. (Tokyo, Japan: Charles E. Tuttle Co., Inc.) Reprinted by permission of the publisher.

Alfalfa

(Medicago sativa; fabacea; LEGUMINOSAE.)

Leaves: Long, slender, serrated at top half; lanceolate; dark green; trifoliate; petioled; mucronate tip.

Stem: Height to 1 m (3 ft.) when erect; sometimes sprawled; slender, lightly furrowed stipules for a sheath; covered with minute downy hairs.

Flowers: Small, delicate, papilonaceous, with five petals; dense, short, terminal clusters; violet or purple.

Fruit: Legume; elongated into two to three spirals containing several olive green seeds; fuzzy pods.

Root: Taproot 15-50 m (20-70 ft.) long; coarse; numerous side branches.

Taste: Young plants are very mild and like sweet lettuce; mature plants are very bitter and grass-like.

Odor: Grass-like.

Part used: Fresh shoots and sprouts of very young plants; dried leaves of the mature plant.

Habitat: This plant is a perennial, extensively cultivated in most temperate parts of the world. It grows in warm, sunny, open areas and is easily recognizable by its bright violet flowers. Alfalfa sprouts are easily grown in glass jars for the eternal fresh salad.

Herbal Use

Alfalfa leaves and sprouts have been used in Mid- and Far Eastern countries for over two thousand years, where the plant is cultivated as a food and a medicine. Only in the last decade has it come to the attention of North Americans for its nutritive value. It contains every vitamin known to man and is a source of calcium, magnesium, phosphorous, aluminum, iron, sulphur, sodium, copper, chlorine, potassium and silicon. Alfalfa also contains many organic salts.

The roots of this plant grow to a great depth, which allows nutrients from many soil levels to be absorbed.

The green leaf of the alfalfa plant contains many enzymes, which are balanced to act on protein, fats, starches and sugars in the human body.

Medical science has also found triterpene sapogenins in alfalfa which have been proven to be very useful in eliminating arthritis. Other plants containing these triterpene sapogenins are:

- licorice *(Glycyrrhiza glabra)*
- ginseng *(Panax quinquefolium)*
- beech *(Fagus silvatica)*
- English ivy *(Hedera helix)*
- pokeweed *(Phytolacca americana)*
- chickweed *(Stellaria media)*

Juice from the alfalfa plant sweetens the stomach by preventing the growth of putritive bacteria, and indirectly aids the manufacture of B_{12} and beneficial flora. The raw juice also contains magnesium, while the heme pigment contains iron as its central atom. Chlorophyl is nature's major blood-building element for all humans and animals that eat green plants. It activates thirty enzymes in the body and takes a role in the metabolism of protein, fat and carbohydrates.

The fresh juice of the alfalfa plant, which contains crude chlorophyl, has proven effective in removing arthritis, anaemia, protein deficiency and hemorrhage. It is also useful in other disorders such as sinusitis, nervous condition, bone disease, varicose veins, skin infection, pyorrhea, T.B., heart disease, duodenal and gastric ulcers and emphyzema. The herb works both topically and internally with excellent results. A poultice made of fresh alfalfa will make moles and skin growths disappear. Many of these healings have been accomplished in one to three months without any major change in diet. Treatment was, in some cases, carried on from four to eleven months *to complete and sustain the healing.*

A grass and vegetable, alfalfa is absolutely nontoxic. It can be taken over a long period of time without producing harmful side effects. Alfalfa juice is a powerful beverage because of its high nutritive and enzyme content and sets off an immediate reaction within the body, which may show up as nausea or a mild stomach disturbance. Once the body is in a cleaner or more healed state these reactions will disappear. Many doctors try to cure the symptom, which is actually only the body's reaction as it tries to clean itself. In removing a disease, the body may re-experience all the pain and discomfort of the original disease.

Drinking alfalfa juice will bring a number of rewards. Alfalfa juice is a blood cleanser and causes uric acid accumulation to be quickly removed. Used regularly, it works as a healer in many conditions. The old malfunctioning cells will begin to be replaced by new cells until the old cells are eventually digested out. Many diets are incomplete, but drinking alfalfa juice can remedy this because of its great nutritional value.

Twenty years ago, experiments were conducted on old rats equivalent in human age to 90 years. Fed with the juice of alfalfa sprouts the rats began to look and act progressively younger. This regeneration of the body was attributed to the auxins in the immature root tip.

Tea No. 1

Especially good for chronic arthritis.

How to prepare the tea:

20 ml (4 tsp.) alfalfa
1 L (1 qt.) water

Add alfalfa to rapidly boiling water. Cover the pot, remove from the heat and let steep for 10-20 minutes. Strain. Add a dash of soya sauce or lemon juice. Store the tea in a cool place.

Amount to use: 250 ml (1 cup) three or four times a day. May be drunk hot or cold.

Tea No. 2

Particularly beneficial for chronic, hemophilic and acute arthritis; lumbago and gout.

Herbal combination:

30 grams (1 oz.) alfalfa
30 grams (1 oz.) burdock root
30 grams (1 oz.) chaparral
7.5 grams (¼ oz.) parsley

How to prepare the tea:

5 ml (1 tsp.) herb mixture
250 ml (1 cup) water

Put herb mixture into rapidly boiling water. Steep for 15-20 minutes. May be sweetened with honey.

Amount to use: Drink 125 ml (½ cup) two or three times a day, either hot or cold.

Tea No. 3

Drink this tea in cases of chronic, menopausal, hemophilic, acute, degenerative or rheumatoid arthritis and lumbago.

Herbal combination:

30 grams (1 oz.) alfalfa
30 grams (1 oz.) burdock root
30 grams (1 oz.) yellow dock *(Rumex crispus)*
30 grams (1 oz.) horse chestnut *(Castanea dentata)*
30 grams (1 oz.) black cohosh
30 grams (1 oz.) chaparral

How to prepare the tea:

1 ml (¼ tsp.) herb mix
250 ml (1 cup) water

Grind all herbs in a mortar until fine. Put herb mixture into boiling water. Let steep 20-30 minutes. May be sweetened with honey or lemon juice. Store in a cool place.

Amount to use: 250 ml (1 cup) one to two times a day. May be drunk hot or cold.

Herbal Capsules (Tea Alternative)

Use the herbal combination of Tea No. 2 or 3.

Put the herbs into a mortar and grind to a fine powder. Put into gelatin capsules.

Amount to use: 1-5 ml (¼-1 tsp.) per day.

Elixir No. 1

Especially helpful for hemophilic, chronic and degenerative arthritis; gout and osteoarthritis.

How to prepare the elixir:

250 grams (1 cup) freshly grown alfalfa sprouts
125 ml (½ cup) water

Put sprouts and water into a blender and blend for a few seconds. Let stand for 15 minutes. Strain through a fine cloth. Add soya sauce for flavour.

Amount to use: 250 ml (1 cup) a day for one week; then increase to 500 ml (2 cups) a day. Drink very slowly.

Elixir No. 2

Especially effective in treating osteoarthritis, gout and rheumatoid and degenerative arthritis.

Herbal combination:

250 grams (1 cup) alfalfa sprouts
Sticks of celery with leaves
1 large comfrey leaf (1 cup)
1 beet (½ cup)
Cloves of fresh garlic

How to prepare the elixir: Chop vegetables finely. Put into a blender and add water. Blend for a few seconds and let stand 15 minutes. Strain and sweeten with honey.

Amount to use: 250 ml (1 cup) a day for the first week. Then increase serving to 500 ml (2 cups) a day. Drink very slowly.

And God said, ''Behold, I have given you every herb bearing seed which is upon the face of all the earth, and every tree in which is the fruit of a tree yielding seed; to you it shall be for meat.

Genesis 1:29

Balm of Gilead, Balsam Poplar

(Populus balsamifera; P. nigra; P. candicans; SALICACEAE.)

Leaves: Ovoid, gradually tapering with pointed apex, serrated edge, net venation; dark green on top, smooth on both sides. Buds are conical, narrow and pointed with closely imbricated scales; brown, shiny; 1-2 cm (½-¾ in.) long and 5-12 mm (¼-½ in.) thick; sticky in spring with fragrant resins (oleo-resin is contained internally).

Trunk: The tree is large and slender, 20-25 m (22-27 yds.) high and about 30-40 cm (12-16 in.) in diameter. Branches are smooth and round with light grey diagonal striations.

Taste: Mild but slightly bitter.

Odor: Very pleasant, like sweet incense.

Part used: Bark, buds.

Habitat: This fragrant-smelling tree is easily identifiable in the springtime when its incense-like fragrance permeates the air. It is very common in temperate climates and is often found growing in groves. Sister plants such as poplars and balms are similar in medicinal value—quaking aspen *(Populus tremuloides)*, for example.

Herbal Use

Balm of Gilead can be used to treat rheumatism, bronchial disorders, kidney and bladder disorders, stomach complaints and eczema.

Tea

Effective in treating a wide variety of ailments: acute, chronic and rheumatoid arthritis; lumbago; muscular rheumatism; neuralgia; neuritis; sciatica and bursitis.

Herbal combination:

30 grams (1 oz.) balm of Gilead (bark or buds)
15 grams (½ oz.) chickweed
15 grams (½ oz.) mullein
15 grams (½ oz.) licorice *(Glycyrrhiza glabra)*

How to prepare the tea:

30 ml (2 tbsp.) herb mixture
1 L (1 qt.) water

Add herbs to rapidly boiling water. Turn down heat. Simmer gently for 20 minutes. Strain through a fine cloth and add honey to sweeten. Store in a cool place.

Amount to use: 125 ml (½ cup) two to three times a day.

Poultice

To make a poultice for swellings, use the herb mixture in the tea recipe above. Pour enough hot water over the herbs to cover them. Let steep for 20 minutes. Spread the herbs onto cotton or flannel cloth and wrap around the affected joint. Put plastic over it and secure with a tie to keep the poultice moist. Leave on overnight.

Herbal Capsules

Use the herbal combination of the tea. Put all the herbs into a mortar and grind to a fine powder. Put into gelatin capsules.

Amount to use: 1-5 ml (¼-1 tsp.) per day.

The doctor of the future will give no medicine but will interest his patients in the care of the human frame in diet, and in the cause and prevention of disease.

Thomas A. Edison

Black Cohosh, Black Snake Root

(Cimicifuga racemosa; Actaea racemosa; RANUNCULACEAE.)

Leaves: Alternate, with long petioles and large compounded leaf-lets 3-6 cm (1-2½ in.) long that are egg-shaped and deeply cleft. Leaves are deep green.

Stem: Simple, slender, smooth, ribbed, 1-2.5 m (3-8 ft.) tall.

Flowers: White, small and numerous in an elongated, delicate, feathery raceme in which the elongated axis bears flowers on short stems in succession toward the apex. Racemes are 20-50 cm (8-20 in.) long; the petal-like sepals fall early. There are numerous two-cleft stamens with long filaments and one to two sessile pistils with broad stigmas. The outer stamens resemble small petals.

Fruit: Small, dry, oval pods with seeds in two rows.

Root: Rhizome, horizontal, large, 2-15 cm (¾-6 in.) long and 1-3 cm (¼-1 in.) thick, hard and knotty. The rhizomes are slightly annulate with circular scars of bud scale leaves and an upper surface with numerous hard, erect, curved branches. Scars show a radiate structure. The scars are dark brown and appear on the surface. Colour is whitish or dark brown. The bark is radiate wood with a light-coloured pith. Roots are cylindrical, obtuselt quadran-gular, only 1-3 mm thick and 3-12 cm (1-5 in.) long, brown or black and longitudinally wrinkled. The internal cortex is thin and brownish.

Powder: Light brown.

Taste: Bitter.

Odor: Very little.

Part Used: Root.

Habitat: Grows in low bush parts of temperate forest areas. The plant flowers between June and September and the fruit appears in autumn. The roots are gathered in early spring and late fall.

Herbal Use

Black cohosh is a female tonic, for use during menstruation and menopause and in childbirth to ease pain and aid in speedy delivery. It has a relaxing effect on the muscular system, tranquilizes and is antispasmodic. The herb also equalizes circulation and is valuable in the treatment of high blood pressure. It is a tonic to the central nervous system, stimulates secretions of the liver and kidney, has a strong effect on the muscular system and is highly prized for its nervine action. Black cohosh is often used for rheumatism and arthritis.

Tea No. 1

Particularly beneficial during menopause.

How to prepare the tea:

5 ml (1 tsp.) black cohosh
250 ml (1 cup) water

Put herb into boiling water. Let steep for 20 minutes. Strain and sweeten with lemon and honey.

Amount to use: 250 ml (1 cup) one to three times a day.

Tea No. 2

For rheumatoid and acute arthritis; also beneficial during menopause.

Herbal combination:

30 grams (1 oz.) black cohosh
30 grams (1 oz.) comfrey
30 grams (1 oz.) raspberry leaves *(Rubus idaeus)*
7.5 grams (¼ oz.) cinnamon *(Cinnamonum zeylandicum)*
15 grams (½ oz.) mullein

How to prepare the tea:

5 ml (1 tsp.) herb mixture
250 ml (1 cup) water

Put the herb into boiling water. Turn off the heat. Cover and let steep for 20 minutes. Strain through a fine cloth and sweeten with honey.

Amount to use: 250 ml (1 cup) one to three times a day.

Herbal Capsules

Herbal capsules can be prepared using the herb combination of Tea No. 2. Grind the herbs and put into capsules.

Amount to use: 1-3 capsules per day.

Blue Flag, Flag Lily, Water Flag

(Iris versicolor, IRIDACEAE.)

Leaves: Lanceolate, long, striate, narrow and overlapped; 1.5-2 cm (½-1 in.) wide and 0.4-0.7 m (1-2 ft.) long; shorter than the stem of the flower; light green.

Stem: Thick, hollow, straight and almost circular; angled on one side, sometimes branching above; 0.6-0.9 m (2-3 ft.) high.

Flowers: Lily-like, large and beautiful. Blue-violet in colour with yellowish or cream markings at the base of the sepals; purple-veined. Six divisions of the perianth are united into a short tube; outer segments are more than 7 cm (2½ in.) long.

Fruit: Capsule. Oblong, with three lobes and two rows of seeds in each cell.

Root: Cylindrical rhizome; horizontal creeping; fleshy annulate. The joints are about 5 cm (2 in.) long and 2 cm (¾ in.) in diameter. The branched main root is 5-20 cm (2-8 in.) long and compressed towards the larger end, where there are a cup-shaped scar and numerous rings of scars above the greyish-brown root endodermis and cortex.

Powder: Brown.

Taste: Acid.

Odor: Slight.

Part Used: Root.

Habitat: This plant is extensively cultivated as a beautiful garden flower. In the Oriental world it is grown as an ornament and a medicine. It requires a rich, loamy soil.

Herbal Use

Blue flag is excellent for stimulating the action of the kidneys, liver and spleen. It is a blood builder and cleaner, heals the lymphatic system, balances the thyroid and is regarded as a longevity tonic. In cases of rheumatism and arthritis, it is especially good for leg and hip problems.

Tea

Particularly good for menopausal, rheumatoid, tuberculous and chronic arthritis. Do *not* use if you have high blood pressure.

Herbal combination:

30 grams (1 oz.) blue flag
30 grams (1 oz.) black cohosh
30 grams (1 oz.) red clover
7.5 grams (¼ oz.) ginseng powder
15 grams (½ oz.) burdock root

How to prepare the tea:

20 ml (4 tsp.) herb mixture
1 L (1 qt.) water

Put herb into boiling water. Turn off the heat and let stand for 2 hours. Strain and sweeten with honey. Store in a cool place.

Amount to use: 250 ml (1 cup) one to three times a day.

This wide earth do we praise,
Expanded far with paths,
The productive, the full-bearing,
Thy mother, holy plant!

From the Angel of Earth, The Essene Gospel of Peace,
translated by Edmond B. Szekely, Book III, pp. 31-32.
(Cartago, Costa Rica: International Biogenic Society)
Reprinted by permission of the publisher.

Buchu

(Barosma betulina, Diosma betulina, B. crenulata, B. serratifolia, RUTACEAE.)

Leaves: Mid-green in colour; glossy; opposite flat; 2.5-3 cm (1-11/8 in.) long; rhomboid-ovate, with a roundish curled apex.

Stem: Woody shrub, 0.3-1.5 m (1-5 ft.) high, with multiple branching young twigs, covered with immersed oil glands. The bark is stiff, angular, smooth and reddish brown or purple tinged.

Flowers: Solitary and pink.

Fruit: Ovate capsule; 0.5 cm (¼ in.) long and 1-2 cm (½-¾ in.) broad; five-seeded; dark brown.

Odor: Aromatic; resembles peppermint.

Taste: Camphoraceous.

Part Used: Leaves.

Habitat: Grows in warm and hot climates; it requires a long growing season. Thrives in sandy to loamy soil in open sunny areas.

Herbal Use

A mild tranquilizer, buchu is excellent for rheumatism and arthritis. It is also effective in healing the bladder and kidneys, disorders of the male urethral tract and menstrual disorders.

Tea

Especially effective in cases of lumbago, gout and chronic and degenerative arthritis.

Herbal combination:

30 grams (1 oz.) buchu
15 grams (½ oz.) parsley
30 grams (1 oz.) cleavers *(Galium aparine)*
30 grams (1 oz.) comfrey

How to prepare the tea:

20 ml (4 tsp.) herbs
1 L (1 qt.) water

Put herb mixture into boiling water. Turn off heat and let stand for 3 hours. Strain and sweeten with honey. Store in a cool place.

Amount to use: 250 ml (1 cup) one to three times a day.

Burdock Root

(Lappa minor; Arctium lappa; COMPOSITAE; Lesser burdock.)

Leaves: Heart-shaped, oblong, large and undulating, rough, fleshy, dentate, petiolate alternate. Leaves are dark green with lighter colour on the undersurface.

Stem: Thick, wide, spreading branches are 0.6-2 m (2-6½ ft.) high and coarse.

Flowers: Dark mauve in colour. The heads are globular with a calyx of imbricated scale; the bracts have multiple hooked extremities for adhering lightly to objects.

Fruit: Burrs: brownish, globoidal and 1-3 cm (½-1¼ in.) broad; of imbricated scale with hooked extremities that adhere to anything.

Root: Perennial; fusiform or spindle-shaped; 0.5-2 cm (¼-¾ in.) thick and 25-80 cm (10-32 in.) long; brownish grey in colour. Externally the root is longitudinally wrinkled. Has annulate crown, somewhat horny fracture. Dark cambium separates the thick outer bark from the yellowish or whitish porous and radiate wood. Hollow centre, or contains white delicate pith-like tissue.

Powder: Light brown.

Taste: The seeds have a pungent taste. The roots are sweet and slightly bitter.

Part Used: First year's growth of roots, leaves and seeds. The root is the most powerful.

Habitat: Grows in weedy places along the wayside and on wasteland. Likes loamy soil rich in nitrogen. A domestic variety that produces very large sweet roots can be easily cultivated in the garden.

Herbal Use

Burdock root has traditionally been considered one of nature's finest blood purifiers. It is soothing to the kidneys, liver and spleen and cleansing to the lymphatic system. Burdock root increases the flow of urine, removes excess fatty tissue and is excellent for rheumatism, sciatica and arthritis.

Burdock root is a wonderful vegetable in taste as well as in its effects. Cut the stalk before the flower opens and remove the outer skin. It can then be eaten raw in salads or boiled or steamed lightly. Burdock root has the delicate taste of winter melon.

In British Columbia, Japanese and Chinese farmers grow a domesticated variety of burdock. In the summer and early autumn these large, long roots can be obtained in Vancouver's Chinatown. The Chinese and Japanese revere this plant highly for its blood-cleaning "spring tonic" effect on the body. Burdock also has the reputation of being an aphrodisiac. You can obtain seeds for this plant at your local Japanese supermarket under the name of Yoboyar Takinogawa. It is easily cultivated in the home garden.

Tea No. 1

Recommended for chronic and menopausal arthritis and gout. The herbal combination may also be used as a poultice for inflamed joints.

Eliminate coffee, tea and cocoa from your diet while using this combination of herbs.

Herbal combination:

Burdock root
Yellow dock *(Rumex crispus)*
Juniper berries
Chickweed
Jamaica ginger

How to prepare the tea: Put 5 ml (1 tsp.) of each of the first three herbs into 1 litre (1 qt.) of boiling water. Simmer gently for 20 minutes. Add 5 ml (1 tsp.) of each of the remaining herbs. Turn off heat and let steep for another 15 minutes. Add water to make up 1 litre (1 qt.). Strain and store in a cool place.

Amount to use: 125 ml (½ cup) two to four times a day.

Tea No. 2

Use for acute, allergic and rheumatoid arthritis.

Herbal combination:

30 grams (1 oz.) burdock root
4 grams (1/8 oz.) golden seal
30 grams (1 oz.) red clover
30 grams (1 oz.) ginger
30 grams (1 oz.) elderberry *(Sambucus canadensis)*

How to prepare the tea:

5 ml (1 tsp.) herb mixture
250 ml (1 cup) water

Mix all herbs together. Put herb mixture into boiling water. Let simmer for 5 minutes. Strain and sweeten with honey. Use yogurt in the diet the same day.

Amount to use: 250 ml (1 cup) one to three times a day. Do not use for more than two weeks.

We praise the healers of the earth,
They who know the secrets of the herbs and
    plants;
To the healers hath the angel of earth
Revealed her ancient knowledge.
The Lord hath created medicines out of the earth,
And he that is wise shall use them,
Was not the water made sweet with wood,
That the virtue thereof might be known?

*From the Angel of Earth, The Essene Gospel of Peace,
translated by Edmond B. Szekely, Book III, pp. 31-32.
(Cartago, Costa Rica: International Biogenic Society)
Reprinted by permission of the publisher.*

Cayenne

(Capsicum minimum; var. C. fastigiatum.)

Leaves: 1.5-4 cm (½-1½ in.) broad and up to 7.5 cm (3 in.) long. Mid-green in colour. Margin entire; oval with long pointed apex; pinnately paired, with terminal leaf.

Stem: About 0.15 cm (1/16 in.) thick; striate; flexible; 1.3-3.6 m (1½-4 ft.) high; bushy.

Flowers: White, yellow or pinkish; small.

Fruit: 1-3 cm (1/2-1 1/5 in.) long; smooth, shiny and brilliant red; chili pepper-like; filled with seeds.

Taste: A very hot and pungent herb.

Odor: Mild, pepper-like, fresh.

Part Used: Fruit.

Habitat: There are over twenty species of this herb, varying from small house plants to shrubs that grow in warm to hot climates of the world. Cayenne is easily cultivated in the home as a beautiful house plant.

Herbal Use

An excellent stimulant, cayenne also has an equalizing effect on the body which causes the blood to circulate normally thus eliminating high blood pressure.

It has proven effective in treating rheumatism, arthritis, excess bleeding, colds, low and high blood pressure, heart problems, stroke and sore muscles.

Herbal Capsules No. 1

Herbal combination:

30 grams (1 oz.) cayenne
15 grams (½ oz.) ginger
7.5 grams (¼ oz.) golden seal

How to prepare the capsules: Put herbs into a mortar and grind to a fine powder. Put into gelatin capsules.

Amount to use: 5-20 ml (1-4 tsp.) a day. Do not use for more than two weeks.

Liniment

Herbal combination:

15 grams (½ oz.) cayenne
15 grams (½ oz.) prickly ash bark
7.5 grams (¼ oz.) peppermint *(Mentha piperita)*

How to prepare the liniment: Put all the herbs into 500 ml (2 cups) of heated olive oil. Let stand for three days. Shake occasionally. Strain through a fine cloth and bottle.

Amount to use: Massage in, morning and evening. Keep in a cool place.

Herbal Capsules No. 2

Add 30 grams (1 ounce) of chaparral to the herbs in the recipe for Herbal Capsules No. 1. Put into a mortar and grind to a powder. Put into gelatin capsules.

Amount to use: Use 5-20 ml (1-4 tsp.) a day. Use yogurt in the diet the same day.

... who satisfieth thy mouth with good things
so that thy youth is renewed like the eagle's.

Psalm 103:5

Chaparral, Creosote Bush, Greasewood

(Larrea tridentata; L. divaricata: ZYGOPHYLLACEAE.)

Leaves: Entire, elliptical, olive green, resinous; appear divergently.

Stem: Evergreen shrub. Erect, light brown, tangle-branched, brittle, leafy, 0.6-3 m (2-10 ft.) long.

Flowers: Small, delicate, bright yellow. Terminal; grow on short racemes.

Fruit: Globose seed capsule; small, white and densely woolly.

Taste: Extremely bitter and disagreeable.

Odor: Very strong.

Part Used: Leaves and stem.

Habitat: This plant is a favourite of the Plains and Southwest Coast Indians. It grows in very warm climates and has a long growing season. It grows in sandy to loamy soil and requires little rainfall. Chaparral is also used by the Hopi in California.

Herbal Use

Chaparral is excellent for rheumatism, arthritis, cancer and urinary disorders. A cell rebuilder, chaparral also benefits the pancreas and lymphatic system. It is good for sore muscles and promotes longevity.

This plant has been known to clear up arthritis and rheumatism problems in one year when used regularly.

Tea No. 1

How to prepare the tea: Add 5 ml (1 tsp.) of dried chaparral leaves into 250 ml (1 cup) of water. Steep for 20 minutes.

Tea No. 2

Use in cases of acute, chronic, degenerative and rheumatoid arthritis and gout.

Herbal combination:

30 grams (1 oz.) chaparral

15 grams (½ oz.) elderberry *(Sambucus canadensis)*
15 grams (½ oz.) chickweed
15 grams (½ oz.) buckbean *(Menyanthes trifoliata)*

How to prepare the tea: Put 25 ml (5 tsp.) of herb mixture into 1 litre (1 qt.) of boiling water. Turn off heat and allow to steep for 3 hours. Strain and sweeten with honey. Bottle and store in a cool place.

Amount to use: 250 ml (1 cup) one to three times daily for one or two months. After this powder (ground chaparral leaves) may be used. This is an excellent tea.

You showed me nutmegs and nutmeg husks,
Ostrich feathers and elephant tusks,
Hundreds of tons of costly tea
Packed in wood by the Cingalee
And a myriad drugs which disagree—
Cinnamon, myrrh and mace you showed,
Golden paradise birds that glowed,
More cigars than a man can count
And a billion cloves in an odorous mount.

John Masefield

Chickweed

(Stellaria media; Alsine media; CARYOPHYLLACEAE.)

Leaves: Opposite and decussate, sometimes cordate; 6-25 mm (¼-1 in.) long; a light, fresh green; ovate; lower leaves petioled and upper leaves sessile; tufted mass.

Stem: Thin, fragile, weak, trailing; 17-50 cm (5-20 in.) long. A distinct line of fine white hairs runs the length of the stem and its many branches.

Flowers: Very tiny and terminal at the axils of leaves. White or yellow, arranged in clusters, with three to seven stamens, cleft petals, long sepals and long petioles.

Fruit: A very tiny capsule yielding many rough, wrinkled, flattened reddish seeds; easily airborne by wind.

Root: The root system is thin, delicate and branched.

Taste: Young plants taste like mild spinach.

Odor: Slight.

Part Used: The whole plant above the ground.

Habitat: Grows prolifically in meadows, gardens, at forest margins and in open areas. Chickweed can be found in cultivated gardens throughout the growing season. Growth ceases in very hot, dry weather. In temperate climates the plant stays green throughout the winter. A native of Asia, chickweed is found in all temperate parts of the world.

Herbal Use

The delicate, trailing chickweed found in your garden is a wonderful salad ingredient, with a mild spinach-like flavour.

Traditionally revered for its healing properties, chickweed is just becoming known by Western medical science for its medicinal value.

It is used for inflammation; stomach ulcers; rheumatism; arthritis; bronchial disorders; kidney, bladder and spleen problems; nervous disorders; colds and tooth decay.

As a poultice, use for swellings, tumors, burns, inflamed eyes and damaged cells. Prevents scars.

Note: For prolonged use, mix chickweed with other healing plants.

Tea No. 1

Especially effective for chronic, degenerative and hemophilic arthritis.

How to prepare the tea:

20 ml (4 tsp.) chickweed
1 L (1 qt.) water

Add chickweed to rapidly boiling water. Cover the pot, remove from the heat and let steep for 10-20 minutes. Strain. Add a dash of soya sauce.

Amount to use: 250 ml (1 cup) three or four times a day. Drink hot or cold. For prolonged use, chickweed should be mixed with other herbs.

Tea No. 2

Beneficial in cases of chronic, tuberculous, degenerative and hemophilic arthritis and gout.

Herbal combination:

30 grams (1 oz.) chickweed
30 grams (1 oz.) alfalfa
30 grams (1 oz.) comfrey
30 grams (1 oz.) coltsfood *(Tussilago farfara)*
15 grams (½ oz.) elderberries *(Sambucus canadensis)*

How to prepare the tea:

20 ml (4 tsp.) herb mixture
1 L (1 qt.) water

Put herb mixture into rapidly boiling water. Turn off heat and let steep 30 minutes. Add 5 drops ginseng extract.

Amount to use: 250 ml (1 cup) two to three times a day.
Note: Do not add ginseng if you have high blood pressure.

Herbal Capsules

Use the herbal combination of Tea No. 2. Put all the herbs into a mortar and grind to a fine powder. Put into gelatin capsules.

Amount to use: 5-20 ml (1-4 tsp.) a day.

Elixir

Recommended for chronic, degenerative and hemophilic arthritis; osteoarthritis and gout.

Herbal combination:

250 grams (1 cup) freshly picked chickweed
1 large fresh comfrey leaf
Several large carrots (about 125 grams or ½ cup)
Several sticks of celery with leaves (about 125 grams or ½ cup)
375 ml (1½ cups) water

How to prepare the elixir: Chop up the vegetables. Put them into a blender and add water. Blend for a few seconds. Let stand 15 minutes.

Amount to use: 250 ml (1 cup) a day for the first week; then increase to 500 ml (2 cups). Leftovers can be heated to boiling point and used as a light soup.

He preferred to know the power of herbs and their value for curing purposes, and heedless of glory, to exercise that quiet art.

Virgil, Aeneid, Book XII-I-356

Comfrey

(Symphytum officinale; BORAGINACEAE.)

Leaves: Decurrent; 8-30 cm (3-12 in.) long; deeply pinnately veined. Dark green in colour. Petioles are long, except on the top leaves which are small and have short petioles. Lower leaves are large and profuse. Mature leaves are covered with hairs which may cause itching.

Stem: Erect, stiff and furrowed; 0.3-1.5 m (1-5 ft.) high and 0.6-1.7 cm (¼-¾ in.) thick; hollow; many stems at base; covered with hairs.

Flowers: White, mauve, or purple; with drooping inflorescence, tubular corolla, short peduncles, five stamens, slender pedicels and a tail-shaped head. Flowers are 1.3-1.7 cm (½-¾ in.) long.

Fruit: Small, shiny; brown or black.

Root: 1.5-2.5 cm (½-1 in.) thick; branched; woody; has dark brown bark but is white internally; very long and spindle-shaped; filled with tasteless juice.

Taste: Like spinach.

Odor: Mild and fresh.

Part Used: Leaves and root.

Habitat: Perennial, grows from May to October in shady, moist areas. It can be found growing along stream beds and under shady groves of deciduous trees. Roots should be collected in the late autumn or in the spring before growth commences and dried at cool temperatures. Leaves may be harvested at any season. Frequent cutting aids the proliferation of this plant. A few large leaves may be taken from a well-cultivated plant every day.

Herbal Use

Comfrey is one of the most amazing herbs in existence. It is widely revered and used in all Mid-Eastern and Eastern countries. It is also extensively cultivated in the United States, South America and the British Isles.

Comfrey contains iron, manganese, calcium, phosphorous, many of the B vitamins and vitamins C and E.

It is used for internal scars, deterioration of tissue, stomach ulcers and disorders, internal bleeding, scarred lungs and lung cancer, broken bones and bone disease, asthma, bronchitis, eczema, varicose veins, skin problems due to sun exposure and wrinkles.

As a poultice it is used for bleeding, cancers, moles, growths, sebaceous cysts, exzema and other skin disorders.

Its regular use is especially good for arthritis because it not only balances the blood (acid/alkaline) but also rapidly breaks down and carries off excess body acids.

Small comfrey leaves make good salads if you chop them very finely. When steamed they are spinach-like and very good with lots of lemon juice and butter. You can also make cream of comfrey soup (a favourite in the B.C. interior).

The roots of the comfrey plant are much stronger than the leaves. When mixed with milder herbs such as chickweed or comfrey leaves, the roots will seal an open wound within hours and an internal stomach ulcer within a few days. Dried roots are good for tea when a critical condition exists or when very powerful healing action is required. Comfrey leaves will work the same but take a little longer, which is often desirable if the person using them is elderly, very ill or not very strong.

Both roots and leaves can be used dry or fresh, although the fresh ones are more powerful.

Tea No. 1

Excellent in cases of osteoarthritis.

How to prepare the tea:

5 ml (1 tsp.) comfrey
250 ml (1 cup) water

Add herb to rapidly boiling water. Turn off heat. Let steep 10 minutes. Strain. Add soya sauce for flavour.

Amount to use: 250 ml (1 cup) one to four times a day.

Tea No. 2

Drink this tea if you have osteoarthritis or degenerative, acute or rheumatoid arthritis.

Herbal combination:

30 grams (1 oz.) comfrey
30 grams (1 oz.) alfalfa

15 grams (½ oz.) chaparral
30 grams (1 oz.) barley *(Hordeum distichun)*

How to prepare the tea:

50 ml (4 tbsp.) barley
20 ml (4 tsp.) herb mixture
1 L (1 qt.) water

Soak barley in water overnight. Boil for 20 minutes. Add herb mixture and turn off heat. Let steep 20 minutes.

Amount to use: 125 ml (½ cup) two to four times a day.

Elixir No. 1

Particularly beneficial for degenerative arthritis and osteoarthritis.

How to prepare the elixir:

250 ml (1 cup) chopped fresh comfrey leaves
250 ml (1 cup) water

Put comfrey leaves into a blender and add water. Blend for a few seconds and then strain through a cloth. Add soya sauce.

Amount to use: 250 ml (1 cup) a day for the first week. Then increase to 500 ml (2 cups) a day. Drink very slowly.

Elixir No. 2

Excellent for osteoarthritis and gout, as well as degenerative and rheumatoid arthritis.

Herbal combination:

2 comfrey leaves (about 250 ml or 1 cup)
1 beet (about 125 ml or ½ cup)
1 clove garlic
1 carrot (about 125 ml or ½ cup)
125 ml (½ cup) chopped lettuce
1 stick celery with leaves (about 65 ml or ¼ cup)

How to prepare the elixir:

250 ml (1 cup) chopped vegetables
250 ml (1 cup) water

Put water and vegetables into blender.

Amount to use: 250 ml (1 cup) a day for the first week, then increase to 500 ml (2 cups) a day.

Corn Silk, Maize, Indian Corn

(Stigmata maydis L. var. rugosa, GRAMINEAE.)

Leaves: Lanceolate, with a long and slender apex; up to 60 cm (25 in.) long on a mature plant. Many of the leaves are wrapped around the fruit. Outer leaves are dark green; inner leaves are light green. Leaves are lightly and closely furrowed and clasping around the base.

Stem: Tall, straight, up to 3.5 m (8 ft.) high, hollow, thick and strong.

Fruit: Cob. Yellow kernels grow in longitudinal lines and are closely packed.

Root: Roots are fibrous with smaller prop roots near the ground.

Flower: Staminate flowers are in tassels at the top of plant; pollen is windblown to "silk" on tip of pistil in "ear" lower on plant.

Taste: Very mild and sweet.

Part Used: Silk at top of mature cob.

Habitat: Cultivated extensively in all rural areas in large fields; an annual.

Herbal Use

Corn silk has long been used by the Indians of the Canadian West Coast and the Mid- and Western United States for all forms of arthritis, stomach complaints and kidney and bladder problems.

It quickly removes an unbalanced condition in the blood caused by the buildup of phosphoric or uric acid. It solves high blood pressure, cholesterol and arteriosclerosis problems.

In sweet corn the sugars are not changed to starches at the immature stage, so the kernels remain sweet and can be prepared when still green. Corn is a good source of calcium, phosphorus, iron, protein and vitamins A and B.

This herb is very easily utilized in the diet by adding the silk to soups and stews, where it provides wonderful flavour and acts as a thickener. As a tea it is delicious, especially if other herbs such as mint or anise are added.

Elixir No. 1

Herbal combination:

Corn silk from ears of 6 corn
8 large shiitake mushrooms
Green onions
Soya sauce

How to prepare the elixir: Put shiitake into 2 litres (2 qts.) boiling water. Boil gently for 1 hour. Remove the mushrooms from the liquid. Add corn silk and simmer at very low heat for 20 minutes. Remove the stems from the mushrooms and chop the caps very finely. Add mushrooms to the broth. Top with finely chopped onions. Delicious.

Amount to use: Eat a large bowl as often as you like.

Accuse not nature, she hath done her part;
Do thou but thine.

John Milton, Paradise Lost

Dandelion

(Taraxacum officinale; Taraxacum dens-leonis; COMPOSITAE.)

Leaves: 5-25 cm (2-10 in.) long and oblong in shape; pinnate; coarsely toothed; shiny; runcinate; rosette near the ground.

Stem: Slender, smooth and straight; flexible, with soft, downy hairs on surface; bears a single head of yellow flowers. Milky juice exudes from broken stems.

Flowers: Brilliant yellow, with a hollow peduncle and heads composed of multiple small florets. The corolla has five teeth; contains a single ovule; opens in the morning and closes at night.

Fruit: 6 mm (¼ in.) long; light brown; radially plumed.

Root: Long, thick taproot; blackish brown outside and whitish inside; can be simple or branched. The roots are fleshy and brittle and exude milky juice when broken. Older roots are divided at the crown.

Taste: Slightly bitter.

Odor: Mild.

Part Used: Leaves and roots.

Habitat: This is one of the first flowers to bloom profusely in the early spring. It can be found in the open areas of forests, meadows and pasturelands. It grows throughout the growing season into the late fall. Dandelions are natives of Eurasia. The leaves make an excellent potherb and wine can be prepared by fermenting the flowers.

Herbal Use

The dandelion was used medicinally long before 300 B.C., when it was first described by Theophastus. It was a common medicine to the early Egyptians, and has been cultivated as a medicine in the Orient for centuries.

Both dandelion leaves and roots are highly prized as medicine. They contain insulin, taraxin, gluten, gum potash and sugars. Insulin occurs in the cell sap and in the root appears as a transparent solid. The leaves contain 75,000 units of vitamin A per ounce, large amounts of the B vitamins, vitamins C and G and others. They also contain iron, calcium, phosphorus and an abundance of minerals. The sodium and other elements which occur naturally in the leaves purify and balance the blood, removing excess uric acid.

The dandelion is especially beneficial for urinary, kidney and liver disorders. It is also used to treat rheumatism, arthritis, stomach disorders, eczema and skin problems.

The roots of the dandelion should be gathered in the autumn. Choose plants which are at least three years old. They may be dried and toasted for use during the winter or kept buried in soil.

Tea No. 1

Use for chronic and degenerative arthritis and gout.

Herbal combination:

30 grams (1 oz.) dandelion root (toasted)
30 grams (1 oz.) ginger
30 grams (1 oz.) chaparral
15 grams (½ oz.) licorice *(Glycyrrhiza glabra)*
5 drops ginseng extract

How to prepare the tea:

5 ml (1 tsp.) herb mixture
250 ml (1 cup) water

Put mixture into water and simmer for 5 minutes. Sweeten with honey. Excellent.

Amount to use: 250 ml (1 cup) one to three times a day.

Tea No. 2

Especially beneficial for acute, degenerative and rheumatoid arthritis and gout.

How to prepare the tea:

250 ml (1 cup) fresh dandelion leaves, chopped
Salted water
250 ml (1 cup) water

Soak leaves in salt water for ½ hour. Rinse. Put dandelion leaves in 1 cup boiling water and let steep 20 minutes.

Amount to use: 250 ml (1 cup) two to three times a day.

Elixir No. 1

Beneficial in cases of acute, degenerative and rheumatoid arthritis and gout.

How to prepare the elixir:

250 ml (1 cup) small spring dandelion leaves and roots, chopped
Salted water and fresh water
500 ml (2 cups) water

Put leaves into cold saltwater and let soak for 1 hour. Rinse well and then soak another ½ hour in fresh water. This removes the bitterness. Put leaves into a blender, add water. Blend for a few seconds. Strain through a fine cloth.

Amount to use: Drink 250 ml (1 cup) a day for the first week. Increase to 500 ml (2 cups) the second week. Drink very slowly.

Elixir No. 2

Effective in treating acute, degenerative and rheumatoid arthritis; osteoarthritis and gout.

Herbal combination:

500 ml (2 cups) spring dandelion leaves
1 large comfrey leaf (about 125 ml or ½ cup)
1 large carrot (about 125 ml or ½ cup)
1 clove garlic

How to prepare the elixir:

250 ml (1 cup) chopped vegetables
Salted water
250 ml (1 cup) water

Rinse freshly picked leaves and soak in saltwater for 1 hour. Put all herbs and vegetables into a blender, add water and blend for a few seconds. Strain through a cloth or put through a juicer.

Amount to use: Drink 250 ml (1 cup) a day for the first week. Increase to 500 ml (2 cups) a day. Drink very slowly.

"Coffee"

Excellent for chronic arthritis and gout.

How to prepare the coffee:

5 ml (1 tsp.) toasted dandelion root
250 ml (1 cup) water

Simmer gently for 5 minutes. Strain. Add honey to sweeten.

Amount to use: Use instead of coffee.

Garden Carrot

(Oxheart CHANTENEY NANTES: UMBELLIFERAE.)

Leaves: Tiny and oval with a pointed apex; in a feather-like grouping; unpaired; dark green.

Stem: 15-30 cm (6-12 in.) high and 1.5-3 mm (1/16-1/8 in.) thick; flexible; light green. The stems grow in clusters on top of the taproot.

Root: Taproot, 1.25-7.5 cm (½-3 in.) thick and 15-37.5 cm (6-15 in.) long; fleshy, with vertical striations. Colour is bright orange with a lighter central core.

Taste: Sweet and mild.

Odor: Fresh.

Part Used: Root and leaves.

Habitat: Internationally cultivated in the home garden.

Herbal Use

A tonic and blood cleanser, the carrot is used herbally to treat not only rheumatism and arthritis, but also eye weakness, cancer, digestion problems, anemia and skin disorders.

When included in the diet, carrots are beneficial for all forms of arthritis.

Elixir

Recommended especially for chronic and rheumatoid arthritis and gout.

How to prepare the elixir: Put equal amounts of carrots (use only organically grown carrots) and celery through a juicer; or, put into a blender and add sufficient water to mix, then strain through a fine cloth.

Amount to use: Drink 250 ml (1 cup) a day, up to three or four cups a week. Drink very slowly. Do not use every day or for a prolonged period of time.

Garlic

(Allium sativum; LILIACEAE.)

Leaves: Long, delicate, narrow, flat and wheat-like.

Stem: Simple, erect and grows from the bulb. Has sheathed leaves and single terminal flowers with umbel above.

Flowers: Globular terminal umbel containing small white flowers, gathered together, with white membranous bract surrounding them.

Bulb: Subglobular, 3-5 cm (1-2 in.) broad. Is a compound of 8-15 bulblets or cloves held together by a white membrane or skin. This membrane forms a sac and is attached to a flattened circular base which has numerous yellowish-white roots. Each clove is delicately covered by the membrane. There is an underlying white, pinkish or purple epidermal layer which coheres but is easily separable from the solid portion.

Taste: Sweet to hot; onion-like but much stronger.

Odor: Very pungent.

Part Used: Bulb and leaves.

Habitat: Garlic is cultivated in the garden in most parts of the world. White garlic is grown in hot southern climates and is very mild and sweet, while the purple-skinned variety grown in temperate and northern cimates tends to be stronger and more pungent. Garlic is easily cultivated indoors for the greens and outdoors for the bulbs.

Herbal Use

In ancient times garlic was used both in healing and for nutrition as it was known to contain great resources for physical strength and energy. It is a valuable nervine and is especially useful in lowering hypertension. Garlic also equalizes blood circulation. It is effective in arresting intestinal putrefaction and infection while stimulating the healthful growth of friendly bacteria. It is also known as "Russian penicillin."

Garlic can be prepared as a drink, applied externally as an ointment and used as a poultice. The small cloves can be swallowed whole.

Garlic is especially beneficial for those who have rheumatoid and acute arthritis. In cases of acute arthritis, combine garlic with any tea containing lobelia or golden seal.

Garlic Oil

How to prepare the oil:

454 grams (1 lb.) garlic
Warm olive oil

Crush garlic and pour olive oil over it. Shake and allow to stand for 2-3 days. Strain through a fine cloth. Bottle and keep in a cool place.

Amount to use: Take one small spoonful three times a day, or use liberally on salads and vegetables.

Fresh Garlic

White sweet garlic may be peeled and eaten raw. Eat 1-3 small cloves per day. Parsley tea, which contains chlorophyl, will neutralize the smell. A clove or two of garlic makes a wonderful addition to any of the elixirs. Do not use every day or for a prolonged period of time.

O mickle is the powerful grace that lies
In herbs, plants, stones, and their true qualities.

Romeo and Juliet II, iii.

Ginseng

(Panax repens, var. Panax pseudoginseng, Ginseng quinquefolium; ARALIACEAE.)

Leaves: Compounded. Three to five large, single leaves 5-12 cm (2-5 in.) long are found on each stem branch. Leaves are obovate-oblong and have serrated edges and a pointed apex. Colour is mid-green. The plant develops a solitary bud at the crown which produces leaves and a stem for the next year; the bud alternates its position on the stem from right to left each year. Leaves appear at intervals along the rhizome.

Stem: Slender, straight. Height varies from 10-20 cm (4-8 in.) to 40-50 cm (16-20 in.), depending on the age of the plant. Colour is mid-green changing to dark green by the end of the season. Branches are smooth; the stem produces 3 or 4 small green branches.

Flowers: In the fourth year of growth a pale green flower cluster forms on the top. Flowers have 5 pointed petals.

Fruit: Round green berries the size of a cherry pit which turn bright crimson in maturity. Fruit grows in the cluster before the new leaves unfold. In British Columbia the berries are dark purple.

Roots: Rhizome, light beige, very fleshy and sweet, large and sometimes forked, generally fusiform. Root often takes human forms. Every year the greenery dies and leaves a growth ring or scar at the neck of the root. Age can be defined by these markings.

Habitat: This herb is cultivated extensively throughout the Orient and North America. In the wilderness it can be found growing on the north side of forested mountains at elevations over 2,500 ft. *Note: Panax repens* is extensively cultivated in China and Japan. *Ginseng quinquefolium* grows in Canada and the United States. The Oriental species of this plant is more potent than that in North America; however, both contain many of the same healing properties.

Herbal Use

A tonic, ginseng improves health and promotes longevity. It is a useful addition to any rheumatism or arthritis healing program.

Ginseng may be taken in capsule or powder form or mixed with tea. Do not use it if you have high blood pressure. Red ginseng is reserved for those over 50 years as it contains many additional medicines.

Ginseng Essence

Cook dried ginseng root until only a fine sediment or paste remains. This usually takes from 16 to 20 hours. Store in a glass jar with a plastic top.

Ginseng Powder

To improve digestion, eat 1 ml (¼ tsp.) of ginseng powder—the ground, powdered root—two times a day.

Tea No. 1

For improving the circulation.

How to make the tea: Combine a small quantity of ginseng essence (see instructions above), no more than 2-5 drops, with water for tea.

Amount to use: Drink one cup two times a day.

Tea No. 2

For stiffness.

Herbal combination:

1 part ginseng essence
1 part mugwort, also called wormwood *(Artissima vulgaris)*

How to make the tea: Use 1 ml (¼ tsp.) herb mixture per 250 ml (1 cup) boiling water.

Amount to use: Drink 1 cup three times a day.

Tea No. 3

Excellent for very old people.

Herbal combination:

5 ml (1 tsp.) strong ginger tea
5 ml (1 tsp.) honey
1 ml (¼ tsp.) ginseng root (powdered)
Water in which rice has been boiled

How to make the tea: Add the first three ingredients to 250 ml (1 cup) of rice water.

Ginseng Extract

Three drops of ginseng extract (which you can purchase from a herb shop) can be added to your favourite herbal tea.

Note: Do not use ginseng if you have high blood pressure.

The Artharva-Veda XI, iv, To the Breath of Life (Prama)

15.

The Breath of Life some call the wind
   (matarisvam);
Again it's caused the breeze *(vata)*.
In the breath of life is what is past and what is
   yet to be;
On the Breath of Life all things are based.

16.

Atharvan plants, Angiras plants, plants derived
   from gods or men,
O Breath of Life, are born when thou dost
   quicken them.

17.

When the Breath of Life this mighty earth with
   rain bedews
The plants are born, whatever herbs there are.

Hindu Scriptures, p. 29. (Toronto, Ontario: J.M. Dent and Sons (Canada) Ltd.) Reprinted by permission of the publisher.

Golden Seal

(Hydrastis canadensis; RANUNCULACEAE.)

Leaves: 5-10 cm (2-4 in.) long and 10-25 cm (4-10 in.) broad; lobed; palmately cleft, with a serrate margin and deep radiate venation. Minute hairs cover the leaf surface. There are usually only 2-3 leaves on a stem. Unequal terminal leaves die soon after the fruit ripens.

Stem: 13-17 cm (5-27 in.) long and 0.2-0.6 cm (1/16-1/4 in.) thick; purplish; hairy. There are several stems to a common rootstalk.

Flowers: Small; greenish white or pink; only one per stem.

Fruit: One bright red berry which looks like a large raspberry; contains 20-25 blackish seeds.

Root: Rhizome; up to 5 cm (2 in.) long and 2.5 cm (1 in.) thick; fleshy; yellowish in colour. Rootlets are profuse and are covered with yellowish hairs.

Taste: Very bitter and acrid.

Odor: Disagreeable.

Part Used: Root.

Habitat: Grows in the rich humus of deciduous forests and on the northern slopes of ravines. Golden seal is cultivated in herb farms in North America and the Orient, but most of the herb in use has been gathered in the wilderness. Plants should be harvested in the autumn. This plant grows in a similar environment to that of ginseng.

Herbal Use

Golden seal is one of the most powerful healers in the herbal kingdom and is used extensively in herbal combinations.

Golden seal was widely used by the Indians of both Canada and the United States for a variety of purposes. It was considered a fine herbal cure-all and was also used for dyeing cloth a brilliant yellow colour.

Besides being an excellent healer of rheumatic pain, golden seal has much else to recommend it.

The leaves of this plant contain a rapid healing agent which will quickly heal open wounds and bruises.

For eye problems, there is no herb comparable to golden seal root. Prepared as a cold infusion and used as an eyewash along with an internal drink, this herb will remove any eye inflammation and soothe any pain in the area.

Golden seal also works quickly to remove any external inflammations or infections. For skin conditions such as acne and eczema a golden seal wash is extremely effective. For nervous rashes and itchiness of the skin a mild wash of the root will provide immediate relief.

Golden seal works well for all disorders of the stomach, correcting bowel complaints and irritation of the mucus membrane.

Golden seal is used as a remedy for still other complaints: ear inflammation; diseases of the eustachian tubes, pharynx, urethra, vagina and uterus; hemorrhoids; sporiasis; boils; bladder problems and cancer. It acts as a tonic to the heart, blood and kidneys.

When golden seal is taken internally or applied topically, large amounts of mucus start to expell. This is due to its stimulating action on the blood capillaries. Because it is so powerful, golden seal should be used internally in very small quantities.

Do not use this herb for a prolonged period of time. If you have high blood pressure, *do not* take golden seal at all, as it could overstimulate the central nervous system.

Tea No. 1

Herbal combination:

15 grams (½ oz.) golden seal
15 grams (½ oz.) mullein
15 grams (½ oz.) echinacea *(Echinacea augustifolia)*
30 grams (1 oz.) comfrey
30 grams (1 oz.) red clover

Put all herbs into a mortar and mix well.

How to prepare the tea:

2 ml (½ tsp.) herb mixture
250 ml (1 cup) water

Simmer for 5-10 minutes. Strain through a fine cloth.

Amount to use: Use one to two cups a day. Do not use longer than one week at a time.

Tea No. 2

Herbal combination:

15 grams (½ oz.) golden seal
60 grams (2 oz.) chickweed
30 grams (1 oz.) comfrey
15 grams (½ oz.) mullein

How to prepare the tea:

5 ml (1 tsp.) herb mixture
250 ml (1 cup) water

Combine herb mixture and boiling water and let steep for 7-10 minutes.

Amount to use: Drink one small cup twice a day. Use yogurt in your diet the same day. Do not use tea for longer than 2 weeks.

Herbal Capsules No. 1

Grind 30 grams (1 oz.) of golden seal and put into capsules.

Take 2-4 #00 capsules per day. Use yogurt in your diet the same day. Do not take for longer than 2 weeks.

Herbal Capsules No. 2

Grind the herbs in the Tea No. 1 recipe into a fine powder and put into #00 capsules.

Take 3-4 capsules a day. Use yogurt in your diet the same day. Do not use longer than one week at a time.

Gotu Kola

(Centella Asiatica, Hyrocotyle Asiatica,
HYDROCOTYLOIDEAE, UMBELLIFERAE.)

Leaves: Small (1-4 cm or ⅓-1½ in.), smooth, shiny and round. Petiolate, undulating, cleft at stem, crenate, with palmate venation and radial attachment to stem. Colour is light green.

Stem: A long, slender, flexible, sprawling vine which creeps along the ground.

Flowers: Small; white or greenish-white.

Root: Taproot; light beige, with many small and fragile branches.

Taste: Mild.

Powder: Green.

Part Used: Fresh and dried leaves.

Odor: Mild and fresh.

Habitat: A member of the violet family, with over 70 subspecies, gotu kola grows in open, sunny areas with lots of moisture. It is easily cultivated as a house plant.

Herbal Use

Gotu Kola has been used in India, China and Japan for centuries, and is familiar to the North American Indian as a healing plant close in value to ginseng.

This plant will help the body return to a healthy condition and will eliminate disorders like rheumatism, nervous breakdown and a variety of other ailments if it is used daily and the body is exposed to the sun.

Gotu kola is used in Oriental medicine for its specific action on the nervous system and brain. It is a blood purifier, used for inflammation, infections and liver, spleen and kidney disorders. It is also a general health tonic.

Gotu kola will stimulate the mind after a short period of regular use, stimulate and improve the memory, give great amounts of physical vitality, reduce stress responses and greatly increase the normal life span.

This plant has often been confused with *Fo-ti-tieng,* the

legendary longevity panacea. Gotu kola is merely a component of this commercially prepared blend.

It is best to use gotu kola fresh, as in salads, or to ingest the herb in capsule form. Teas made from this herb will not do as much good as will using the whole fresh herb, but many of the fine qualities attributed to gotu kola will shine forth anyway. Gotu kola will act beneficially in any healing program.

This plant can be cultivated indoors as a house plant or put in the garden if climate permits.

Tea No. 1—Good Health Tea

Herbal combination:

30 grams (1 oz.) gotu kola
30 grams (1 oz.) comfrey
4 grams (1/8 oz.) ginseng powder
4 grams (1/8 oz.) licorice *(Glycyrrhiza glabra)*

How to prepare the tea:

5 ml (1 tsp.) herb mixture
250 ml (1 cup) water

Pour boiling water over the herb mixture. Let steep for 10 minutes.

Amount to use: Use 1-3 cups a day and stay in the sun for an hour.

Tea No. 2—Longevity Tea

Herbal combination:

15 grams (½ oz.) malva flowers *(Malva sylvestris)*
30 grams (1 oz.) gotu kola leaves
30 grams (1 oz.) raspberry leaves *(Rubus idaeus)*
30 grams (1 oz.) comfrey
5 ml (1 tsp.) cinnamon *(Cinnamonum zeylandicum)*

How to prepare the tea:

5 ml (1 tsp.) herb mixture
250 ml (1 cup) water

Pour boiling water over the herb mixture. Let steep for 7-10 minutes.

Amount to use: Use as often as you like, drinking about 250-750 ml (1-3 cups) a day. Stay in the sun for an hour.

Hops

(Humulus lupulus; CANNABINACEAE:
MORACEAE URTICACAE.)

Leaves: Opposite, deep green, very rough, 3-5 lobed, serrated, and with a cordate venate or veined stalk.

Stem: Long and twining, with several rough and angular flexible stems. The stem is up to 6 m (6½ yds.) long and will grow around any adjacent support.

Flowers: Male and female plants with numerous greenish pistils, cone-like spikes which produce fruit.

Fruit: Strobiles or catkins, ovoid cylindrical, round, 2-4 cm (1-1½ in.) long with multiple yellow-green scales that overlap each other. The fruit has numerous brown glandular hairs, lupulin, at the base of each scale and enclosing a glandular achene.

Taste: Aromatic, slightly astringent and exceedingly bitter.

Odor: Sweet, fresh, strong. Upon cutting the fruit the odor becomes disagreeable, resembling that of valerian.

Part Used: Fruit.

Habitat: Hops is a common high-fence plant in moderate climates. It is easily cultivated.

Herbal Use

Hops is very stimulating and functions as a nerve tonic. It increases the flow of urine and can, over a period of time, dissolve solidified calculi. It is a mild pain killer. Hops is used to heal rheumatism and inflammations.

Tea

Particularly beneficial in cases of chronic, degenerative and rheumatoid arthritis; lumbago and gout.

Herbal combination:

30 grams (1 oz.) hops
30 grams (1 oz.) comfrey
7.5 grams (¼ oz.) Jamaica ginger

15 grams (½ oz.) elderberries *(Sambucus canadensis)*
15 grams (½ oz.) peppermint *(Mentha piperita)*

How to prepare the tea:

20 ml (4 tsp.) herb mixture
1 L (1 qt.) water

   Put boiling water over herb mixture. Let stand for half an hour. Store in a cool place.

Amount to use: Drink 250 ml (1 cup) one to three times a day.

One may heal with goodness,
One may heal with justice,
One may heal with herbs,
One may heal with the Wise Word.
Amongst all the remedies
This one is the healing one
That heals with the Wise Word,
This one it is that will best drive away sickness
From the bodies of the faithful,
For wisdom is the best healing of all remedies.

From the Angel of Wisdom, The Essene Gospel of Peace,
translated by Edmond B. Szekely, Book III, p. 51.
(Cartago, Costa Rica: International Biogenic Society)
Reprinted by permission of the publisher.

Jamaica Ginger, Ginger

(Zingiber officinale: ARISTOLOCH.)

Leaves: Entire and reed-like, with a pointed apex, longitudinally striated venation, mid-green, 0.3-0.6 m (1-2 ft.) long. The plant develops a large globular capsule-like form at the crown on which the flowers grow.

Stem: 0.6-1.5 m (2-5 ft.) tall, thick and fleshy, consisting of many overlapping leaves. Light green.

Flowers: 6-10 cm (2½-4 in.) across, a light whitish-green and fragrant; the flowers appear on the crown on a capsule. Three to four flowers grow singly at various intervals.

Roots: Thick, fleshy, annulate and sweet. The horizontal rhizome segments are a golden light brown, with a surface stem scar and yellow interior.

Taste: Sweet and pungent, very aromatic.

Odor: Fragrant.

Habitat: This plant grows in semi-tropical and tropical climates but is easily cultivated as a house plant.

Herbal Use

Ginger is excellent for healing rheumatism. The plant is used for cooking and as a beverage. It has a warming effect in winter and a cooling effect in summer.

Tea

Recommended especially for chronic arthritis.

How to prepare the tea:

20 ml (4 tsp.) chopped ginger root
250 ml (1 cup) water

Pour boiling water over ginger. Steep for 10 minutes. Add lemon.

Amount to use: Drink 250 ml (1 cup) three to four times a day.

Juniper Berry

(Juniperis communis; PINACEA var. saxatilis.)

Leaves: Grow in narrow whorls of three, 8-12 mm (⅓-½ in.) long, have sharp points, are concave and lanceolate and have silver bands of stomata above.

Trunk: Sprawling shrub (only rarely a tree) with its main limbs 2-5 m (6½-16 ft.) long, some of which are often found near the ground. There are many close branches.

Fruit: Berries, which are globular and 5-9 mm (1/5-1/3 in.) in diameter and have a blue-grey waxy covering. Three bracts form the fruit, which contains 3 ovate seeds.

Powder: Dark brown.

Odor: Aromatic.

Taste: Sweet and pleasant, then bitter.

Part Used: Berries and oil from the wood.

Habitat: Juniper is found all along ocean coast areas and in mountainous areas up to the frost line. The berries are usually collected in the second year of growth when they have turned a deep blue.

Herbal Use

A blood cleanser, juniper berries can also be used to treat many other ailments: inflamed kidneys; spleen, bladder, urinary, bronchial and nervous disorders; weak stomach; fungus growths and epilepsy. Teas containing juniper berries are often used to treat rheumatoid arthritis and gout.

Tea No. 1

Particularly helpful if you have rheumatoid arthritis or gout.

Herbal combination:

30 grams (1 oz.) juniper berries
15 grams (½ oz.) ginger

30 grams (1 oz.) dandelion root
5 ml (1 tsp.) cinnamon *(Cinnamonum zeylandicum)*

How to prepare the tea:

25 ml (5 tsp.) herb mixture
1 L (1 qt.) water

Pour boiling water over herb mixture and let stand overnight. Strain. Sweeten with honey. Store in a cool place.

Amount to use: Drink 250 ml (1 cup) one to two times a day.

Tea No. 2

Excellent for chronic and rheumatoid arthritis and gout.

How to prepare the tea:

125 ml (½ cup) fresh juniper berries
250 ml (1 cup) water

Pour water over crushed berries. Steep for 10-15 minutes. Strain. Add honey for flavour.

Amount to use: Drink 250 ml (1 cup) two to three times a day.

. . . And the fruit thereof shall be for meat, and the leaf thereof for medicine.

Ezekiel 47:12

Lobelia

(Lobelia inflata: LOBELIACEAE.)

Leaves: Alternate, ovate-lanceolate, oblong, serrate, veiny, hairy and pale green in colour.

Stem: Cylindrical and angular, hairy, 0.15-1 m (6-40 in.) high; a yellowish light green in colour.

Flowers: Numerous, small, bell-shaped and pale blue in colour, positioned on long racemes and with short pedicels.

Fruit: An inflated two-celled oval capsule containing a number of small (0.8-1.5 cm or ⅓-⅔ in. long), ovate-oblong, light brown seeds. These are coarsely reticulated on the outer surface.

Odor: Strong and irritating.

Taste: Strong. Repugnant.

Part Used: Leaves and seeds.

Habitat: This is an open-area weed. It grows in temperate and hot climates in sunny meadows and pastures. It is cultivated in gardens in Asia, the United States and Canada.

Herbal Use

Besides rheumatism and arthritis, lobelia is used to heal many other conditions: epilepsy, convulsions, spasmodic problems and nervous disorders; respiratory problems and asthma; over-worked heart; pain from sprains; inflammation and swellings; hepatitis and brain disorders. It is a tranquilizer, muscle relaxant, poison antidote and blood cleanser.

Tea

A good herbal treatment for almost any arthritic problem: acute, chronic, gonorrheal and rheumatoid arthritis; gout; lumbago; muscular rheumatism; neuralgia; neuritis; sciatica and bursitis.

Herbal combination:

30 grams (1 oz.) lobelia
30 grams (1 oz.) Jamaica ginger
7.5 grams (¼ oz.) yarrow *(Achilles millefolium)*

3 grams (1/10 oz.) golden seal
30 grams (1 oz.) dandelion root
15 grams (½ oz.) licorice *(Glycyrrhiza glabra)*

How to prepare the tea:

20 ml (4 tsp.) herb mixture
1 L (1 qt.) water

Put herb mixture into water and simmer for 20 minutes. Add water to make 1 litre (1 qt.). Store in a cool place.

Amount to use: 250 ml (1 cup) one to two times a day. Use yogurt in your diet the same day.

Poultice for Inflamed Joints

Make a tea from lobelia and Jamaica ginger. Soak a cloth in the tea and apply to the inflamed area.

Nature never did betray the heart that loved her,
'Tis her privilege thru all the years of this
   our life
To lead from joy to joy. For she can so inform
   the mind that is within us, so impress... that all
   which we behold is full of blessings.

William Wordsworth

Mullein

(Verbascum thapsus, Verbasci filia; SCROPHULARIACEAE.)

Leaves: Large, fleshy, soft and velvety, with soft hairs. Pale green. Lower leaves are in a rosette on the ground; the upper ones are lanceolate-oblong and strongly clasp the stem, becoming decurrent, smooth and more ovate in shape, 15-20 cm (6-8 in.) long and 5-6 cm (2-2½ in.) broad. This plant is distinguished from *Verbascum nigrum* and other mulleins in that the leaves narrow at the base into two wings which pass down the stem.

Stem: Thick, straight, simple, 1-1.5 m (3-5 ft.) high, covered with soft woolly fibres with branched hairs.

Flowers: Consist of 5 golden-yellow round petals, 3 cm (1 in.) across; are cup-shaped; are densely situated on a thick woolly spike which is usually more than 30 cm (12 in.) long and is tough, brittle and dry; have 1 pistil and 5 anther-bearing stamens.

Fruit: Capsule or pod.

Taste: Bitter.

Odor: Fragrant.

Part Used: Leaves, flowers, fruit and root.

Habitat: Grows in all temperate parts of the world, in pastures, meadows, waysides and open, sunlit areas of the forest. This is a very beautiful plant and easy to identify.

Herbal Use

Mullein is beneficial in removing internal scar tissue. It is excellent for the respiratory system and a tonic for the pulmonary system. It is an excellent tranquilizer, a pain killer for the nervous system, and it soothes inflamed and irritated areas. Mullein is particularly good for sciatica and inflamed rheumatism and arthritis.

Tea

Recommended for acute, chronic and rheumatoid arthritis; lumbago; muscular rheumatism; neuralgia; neuritis; sciatica and bursitis.

Herbal combination:

30 grams (1 oz.) mullein
30 grams (1 oz.) comfrey
30 grams (1 oz.) raspberry leaves *(Rubus idaeus)*
30 grams (1 oz.) dandelion root
15 grams (½ oz.) Jamaica ginger

How to prepare the tea:

5 ml (1 tsp.) herb mixture
250 ml (1 cup) water

Pour water over herb mixture. Let steep for 15 minutes. Strain through a fine cloth to remove the minute hairs of the mullein leaf.

Amount to use: 250 ml (1 cup) two to three times a day. This tea will help to induce sleep if taken before you go to bed.

Liniment

For stiff joints and rheumatism.

Herbal combination:

60 grams (2 oz.) mullein
30 grams (1 oz.) lobelia
30 grams (1 oz.) white poplar bark
15 grams (½ oz.) Jamaica ginger

How to prepare the liniment: Powder the herbs and place into 1 litre (1 qt.) of hot olive oil. Leave herbs in oil for one week in a warm place. Strain. Rub in after soaking inflamed area in hot water.

All thy garments smell of myrrh, and aloes, and cassia, out of the ivory palaces, whereby they have made thee glad.

Psalms 45:8

Myrrh, Gum Myrrh

(Commiphora myrrha, BURSERACEAE.)

Leaves: Trifoliate, obovate, 2-3 cm (¾-1¼ in.) long. The sessile leaflets are about 1.5 cm (½ in.) long, stalked on short petioles about the size of a pea.

Gum Resin: Rounded, reddish-brown, covered with yellowish dust; irregular tears; waxy fractures; oily and granular.

Trunk: Light.

Odor: Pleasantly agreeable.

Taste: Bitter.

Part Used: Bark, buds and resin.

Habitat: Grows in moderate to very hot climates and is very fragrant-smelling in the spring.

Herbal Use

Myrrh is a stimulant and disinfectant. It has a warming effect, and is used herbally to treat rheumatism, joint inflammation, bronchial disorders, shock, mouth and gum problems and menstrual disorders.

Another camphor tree, *Cinnamonum camphora*, can be used in the same way. It is grown in California as an ornamental tree.

Tea

Particularly beneficial if you have chronic or rheumatoid arthritis, lumbago, sciatica, bursitis, muscular rheumatism, neuralgia or neuritis.

Herbal combination:

30 grams (1 oz.) myrrh powder (bark)
7 grams (¼ oz.) golden seal
30 grams (1 oz.) raspberry leaves *(Rubus idaeus)*
7 grams (¼ oz.) ginger
15 grams (½ oz.) mullein

How to prepare the tea:

5 ml (1 tsp.) herb mixture
250 ml (1 cup) water

Pour boiling water over the herbs. Let steep 10-15 minutes. Strain through a fine cloth. Use yogurt in your diet the same day.

Amount to use: 125 ml (½ cup) two to three times a day. Do not use longer than two weeks at a time.

Poultice

The herb combination listed above makes an excellent poultice for inflamed joints. Soak a cloth in the tea and wrap it around the affected joint.

Zen Prayer for Mealtime

First, seventy-two labours brought up this rice,
We should know how it comes to us.
Second, we should know whether our virtue and
practice deserve it.
Third, as we desire the natural order of the mind,
to be free from clinging, we must be free from
greed.
Fourth, to support our life, we take this food.
Fifth, to attain this way we take this food.

Turning On, by Rasa Gustaitis, p. 160. (New York: MacMillan Publishing Co., Inc.) © 1979 by Rasa Gustaitis. Reprinted by permission of the publisher.

Oregon Grape, Mountain Grape

(Berberis aquifolium; Mahonia aquifolia: BERBERIDACEAE.)

Leaves: Holly-like, with compound shiny leaves which have tough, spine-bearing teeth; thick; ovate; acute; petiolate; dentate. There are 5-7 leaflets per branch.

Stem: A low shrub, the Oregon grape's stem is glaborous, smooth and yellow-grey outside and yellow inside.

Flowers: An elongated cluster with yellowish-green racemes.

Fruit: Bluish-purple berries which look like small grape clusters. The pulp is acrid and the berries contain numerous seeds.

Root: Long, cylindrical rhizome with branching roots; knotty; tough; hard. The wood is yellowish and the bark is brownish. The root is 4-5 cm (1½-2 in.) thick; the bark is thin (0.5-1 mm thick) and separable into layers. The wood is radiate with a small pith, splits on drying and has a wrinkled, hard fracture.

Powder: Yellow-brown.

Odor: None.

Part Used: Rhizome and roots.

Habitat: This plant is found in open areas of coniferous forests.

Herbal Use

Oregon grape is an excellent blood purifier and liver and kidney stimulant. It promotes digestion and absorption and heals skin tissue. The roots contain berberine, an alkaloid good for menstrual disorders. Oregon grape is also effective against rheumatism, arthritis and internal infections.

Tea

Especially good for chronic and rheumatoid arthritis.

How to prepare the tea:

10 ml (2 tsp.) fresh Oregon grape root
250 ml (1 cup) water

Pour water over freshly grated root. Let steep for 10-15 minutes. Strain.

Amount to use: Drink 250 ml (1 cup) one to three times a day.

89

Parsley

(Carum petroselinum; Apium petroselinum; petroselinum sativum; UMBELLIFERAE.)

Leaves: Wedge-shaped leaves are triangular, with 2-3 pinnate segments, and are irregularly dentate, bright green and curly, with long petioles. There is a basal rosette in the first year, a flowering stem the second.

Stem: Smooth, straight and branched at the top; 25-60 cm (10-24 in.) high.

Flowers: Very tiny, greenish-yellow, in flat-topped umbels with 10-20 florets in each umbel.

Fruit: 0.3 cm (1/8 in.) long; ovoid; dark brown; smooth; ribbed when dry.

Root: Spindle-shaped; parsnip-like; light beige; 8-20 cm (3-8 in.) long and up to 2.5 cm (1 in.) thick; a taproot, slightly branched with few rootlets.

Taste: Strong flavour; pleasant.

Odor: Mild.

Part Used: Whole plant.

Habitat: This plant is cultivated extensively in home gardens as a culinary herb. It is a perennial and can be harvested from March until the heavy frost. For better flavour, harvest this plant before the seeds appear. Parsley is easily cultivated in the kitchen window.

Herbal Use

Parsley has been cultivated for culinary and medicinal uses all over the world for 2,000 years. It contains vitamins A, B, C and E and the minerals calcium, magnesium, phosphorous, chlorine, potassium, iron, sodium and sulfur.

A powerful blood cleanser, parsley is used as the major ingredient in many herbal mixtures. It has a soothing and healing effect on the adrenal and thyroid glands. It is used to heal arthritis, swollen glands, disorders of the spleen, kidneys and bladder, and to remove gallstones. It also breaks down uric acid in the system and generally promotes better health.

Parsley is a very powerful herb and is usually mixed with other herbs for best results.

Tea No. 1

Excellent for gout and chronic and rheumatoid arthritis.

How to prepare the tea:

2 ml (½ tsp.) parsley
250 ml (1 cup) water

Pour boiling water over the herb. Steep for 15-20 minutes. Add soya sauce.

Amount to use: 250 ml (1 cup) one to three times a day.

Tea No. 2

Particularly beneficial if you have chronic or rheumatoid arthritis and gout.

Herbal combination:

7 grams (¼ oz.) parsley
7 grams (¼ oz.) juniper berries
30 grams (1 oz.) celery seed *(Apium graveolens)*
5 drops ginseng extract

How to prepare the tea:

5 ml (1 tsp.) herb mixture
250 ml (1 cup) water

Pour boiling water over herb mixture. Let steep for 20 minutes.

Amount to use: 250 ml (1 cup) one to two times a day.

Elixir No. 1

Good for gout and chronic and rheumatoid arthritis.

Herbal combination:

4 large sprigs parsley (about 125 ml or ½ cup)
1/16th head lettuce (about 125 ml or ½ cup)
1 clove garlic
1 large carrot (about 125 ml or ½ cup)

How to prepare the elixir: Put all ingredients into a blender, add 250 ml (1 cup) water and blend for a few seconds. Let stand for one hour. Strain through a cloth.

Amount to use: 250 ml (1 cup) a day for the first week; then increase to 500 ml (2 cups) a day. Drink very slowly.

Peruvian Bark

(Cinchona calisaya, C. officinalis; CINCHONAE.)

Leaves: Oval with pointed apex, net venation; mid to dark green; evergreen; paired leaves with no terminal leaf on the branch.

Trunk: Bark frequently exfoliates, has a patchy appearance, is reddish tinted and has longitudinal and transverse fissures and cracks. The bark rolls when dry and lichens are found growing on it.

Flowers: Small, whitish pink, campanulate, with numerous terminal axillary clusters. Flowers blossom in spring months.

Odor: Mild.

Taste: Bitter.

Part Used: Bark.

Habitat: Peruvian bark grows in South America and all through the areas of India, Sri Lanka, the Orient and Far East which have a long rainy season. It grows at elevations between 5,000 and 20,000 feet. Most is imported from the Eastern countries. The bark must be gathered when the tree is under 15 years old.

Herbal Use

Excellent for acute rheumatism, Peruvian bark removes pain, stimulates circulation and is a tonic to the nervous system. It is also used to treat bronchitis, dropsy, fevers, flu, colds, malaria, gangrene, hay fever, pneumonia, whooping cough, skin disease and stomach weakness.

Tea No. 1

For inflamed and acute rheumatism.

Herbal combination:

15 grams (½ oz.) Peruvian bark
15 grams (½ oz.) orange peel *(Citrus aurantium)*
5 ml (1 tsp.) cinnamon *(Cinnamonum zeylandicum)*

How to prepare the tea: Simmer the herbs for 15 minutes in 1 litre (1 qt.) of water. Strain.

Amount to use: Drink 1-2 cups of tea a day.

Tea No. 2

For acute or inflamed rheumatism.

15 grams (½ oz.) Peruvian bark
15 grams (½ oz.) ginger
15 grams (½ oz.) echinacea *(Echinacea augustifolia)*
7 grams (¼ oz.) licorice *(Glycyrrhiza glabra)*

How to prepare the tea: Simmer the herbs for 15 minutes in 1 litre (1 qt.) water.

Amount to use: Drink 1-2 small cups a day. Do not use for longer than two weeks at a time.

Herbal Capsules

Both of the recipes listed above can be made into powder and put into capsules.

Amount to use: Take 3-4 capsules a day.

Three pints of dewdrops have been sprinkled over three pints of blossoms on the white bush-clover.

Rhota, A Chime of Windbells, p. 69.

Poke Root, Pokeweed, Scoke

(Phytolacca decandra, P. vulga americana;
CHENOPODIACEAE; PHYTOLACCACEA.)

Leaves: Scattered; alternate; oblong to lanceolate and tapering at both ends; 12-18 cm (5-7 in.) long and 8-10 cm (3-4 in.) broad; smooth on both sides; rich green; entire; petiolate.

Stem: Round, smooth, stout, pithy, erect and branching. Green when young and red or purple toward the end of the summer. The stem is 1-3 m (3-10 ft.) high and about 5 cm (2 in.) in diameter.

Flowers: Numerous and small, about 1 cm (½ in.) across; are in racemes 5-20 cm (2-8 in.) long. A calyx of four to five rounded persistent sepals simulate petals. There is no corolla. The styles are curved and there is a conspicuous green ovary. Flowers are white with a green centre and a pink tint outside.

Fruit: Round berries, which are very juicy, dark purplish and 1 cm (½ in.) thick, hang in large, long clusters from reddened foot stalks. The berries are shiny and have ten seeds and purple-red juice.

Root: Large, cylindrical, 3-8 cm (1-3 in.) thick, frequently fleshy and fibrous; is easily cut or broken; is annulate and longitudinally wrinkled. The root is covered with a thin yellowish-brown or brownish-grey bark and is internally whitish in colour.

Powder: Brownish yellow.

Odor: Slight.

Parts Used: Berries, leaves.

Habitat: Pokeweed was once one of the most common vegetables eaten by the early settlers across Canada and the United States. The young, tender leaves were gathered and then boiled. The roots were traditionally used by the Indians to purify the blood and were often referred to in the writings of early explorers. Pokeweed grows in temperate and hot climates. It likes open, sunny areas in meadows and pastures.

Herbal Use

Excellent for rheumatism and arthritis, pokeweed also has many other uses. A mild tranquilizer and an emetic, pokeweed also increases the flow of urine. It can be taken to heal glandular disorders (particularly an enlarged thyroid); spleen, liver and kidney disorders; tumors and growths; skin, obesity and lymphatic system problems; ulcers and cancer.

Tea

Recommended especially for acute, rheumatoid and chronic arthritis.

Herbal combination:

30 grams (1 oz.) pokeweed leaves
30 grams (1 oz.) elderberries *(Sambucus canadensis)*
30 grams (1 oz.) chickweed
15 grams (½ oz.) buckbean *(Menyanthes trifoliata)*

How to prepare the tea:

5 ml (1 tsp.) herb mixture
250 ml (1 cup) water

Pour boiling water over the herb mixture. Let steep for 20 minutes.

Amount to use: 250 ml (1 cup) one to two times a day.

Zen Prayer to End a Meal

The water with which I wash these bowls tastes
   like ambrosia,
I offer it to the various spirits to satisfy them.

Turning On, by Rasa Gustaitis, p. 160. (New York:
MacMillan Publishing Co., Inc.) © 1969 by Rasa Gustaitis.
Reprinted by permission of the publisher.

Prickly Ash

(Zanthoxylum americanum or Z. clava hirculis or Z. faximeum; RUTACEAE.)

Leaves: Ovate and smooth. The edges have small rounded teeth. Pointed apex, slightly blunted.

Trunk: Spiny shrub, usually 1-4 m (3-13 ft.) high, occasionally to 6 m (19½ ft.). The bark is grey to bluish and prickly, with conical spines 2-15 cm (¾-6 in.) long and 2-5 mm (1/25-1/5 in.) thick. The bark itself is 10-15 mm (½-⅔ in.) thick and is fragmented. The outer part shows green and the inner part yellow. The trunk is alternately branched.

Flower: Small, greenish-white, staminate flowers are in sessile axillary clusters.

Fruit: Small blue-black berries, the size of currants, grow in enclosed grey shells that cluster on the top of the branches. These frequently appear before the leaves.

Part Used: Bark and berries.

Habitat: Grows in Eastern Canada and United States.

Herbal Use

The bark and berries of the prickly ash are used herbally to treat rheumatism and arthritis; skin, liver and bronchial disorders; teeth, mouth and gum problems and asthma. Prickly ash is a mild cardiac stimulant and a mild tranquilizer. It strengthens both the heart and the nervous system.

Tea

Particularly beneficial in cases of chronic and rheumatoid arthritis.

Herbal combination:

30 grams (1 oz.) prickly ash
7 grams (¼ oz.) licorice *(Glycyrrhiza glabra)*
3 grams (1/10 oz.) golden seal

30 grams (1 oz.) comfrey
30 grams (1 oz.) peppermint *(Mentha piperita)*

How to prepare the tea: Put 20 ml (4 tsp.) of a mixture of the first three ingredients into 1 litre (1 qt.) boiling water. Simmer for 20 minutes. Add boiling water to make up 1 litre. Add 2 ml (½ tsp.) of mixture of remaining herbs. Let steep another 10 minutes. Use yogurt in the diet the same day. Bottle and store in a cool place.

Amount to use: 250 ml (1 cup) one to three times a day. Do not use longer than two weeks at a time.

Song IX
The Mountain Spirit (Shan Kuei)

It seems that there is someone over there, in that
    fold of the hill,
Clad in creepers, with a belt of mistletoe.
He is gazing at me, his lips parted in a smile;
Have you taken a fancy to me? Do I please you
    with my lovely ways?
Driving red leopards, followed by stripy civets,
Chariot of magnolia, banners of cassia,
Clad in stone-orchid, with a belt of asarum,
I go gathering sweet herbs to give to the one I
    love.
I live in a dark bamboo grove, where I never see
    the sky;
The way was perilous and hard;
That is why I am late for the tryst.

The Nine Songs, translated by Arthur Waley, p. 53.
(San Francisco, Ca.: City Lights) © 1973 by Arthur Waley.
Reprinted by permission of the publisher.

Red Clover

(Trifolium pratense; PAPILIONACEAE; LEGUMINOSAE.)

Leaves: Pinnately three-foliate. Leaflets are oval or obovate, nearly entire, minutely toothed, sometimes with white *V* markings across the upper surface. Dark green; grow on alternate sides of the stem; sometimes covered with fine white hairs. Long, pointed stipules are attached to the petioles.

Stem: Ascending, 25-60 cm (10-24 in.) high, branching, striated, covered with fine white hairs, flexible. Stipules are pointed and broadly overlapping at the leaf base.

Flowers: 2.5-3.7 cm (1-1½ in.) high and 1.3-2.5 cm (½-1 in.) broad. The inflorescence is a dense, ovoid head of bracted, sessile flowers. The multiple flowers are slender and extended-tubular; five-cleft; pink, red, or purple; sweet-smelling; growing from a very delicate stipule covered with light green veins.

Fruit: Dark brown, kidney-shaped.

Root: Diffusely branched and brown, with a taproot almost as deep as that of alfalfa.

Taste: Slightly acidic and sweet.

Odor: Sweet meadow-like.

Part Used: Young leaves and flowers.

Habitat: Biennial; found on roadsides, waysides and pastures. Red clover may grow in small clusters or may cover an entire field. It is in bloom from mid-spring until late autumn. A native of Europe, it is now cultivated in the United States and southern Canada. It was first cultivated in Spain in the fifteenth century. Fields of sweet red clover are very common in rural and forest margin areas.

Herbal Use

Red clover is a fragrant healer and an excellent blood cleaner and balancer. It contains many minerals and salts and has a very high vitamin content. It also contains lime, silica, potash and phosphoric acid as well as many elements. The juice of the leaf is a natural antiseptic. As a poultice, the leaves heal burns and open wounds of all kinds.

The whole plant is good for arthritis, bronchial disorders, colds, urinary disorders and urethritis and is stimulating to the kidneys. It helps to balance the blood by the rapid removal of uric acid and is healing to the nervous system. Red clover flowers, made into a salve, remove external cancers and growths.

Tea

Excellent for chronic, rheumatoid and tubercular arthritis and gout.

Herbal combination:

30 grams (1 oz.) red clover flowers
30 grams (1 oz.) burdock
30 grams (1 oz.) licorice *(Glycyrrhiza glabra)*
30 grams (1 oz.) fresh ginger
30 grams (1 oz.) comfrey
15 grams (½ oz.) golden seal

How to prepare the tea:

5 ml (1 tsp.) herbal mixture
250 ml (1 cup) water

Pour boiling water over the herb mixture. Allow to steep for 20 minutes. Strain. Use yogurt in the diet the same day.

Amount to use: 250 ml (1 cup) one to three times a day. Do not use longer than two weeks at a time.

Elixir

Particularly beneficial for chronic and rheumatoid arthritis and gout.

Herbal combination:

250 ml (1 cup) freshly picked red clover blossoms
1/8 head lettuce (about ½ cup or 125 ml)
Fresh mint
Lemon juice

How to prepare the elixir: Put herbs into a blender, add 250 ml (1 cup) water and blend for a few seconds. Let stand 15 minutes. Strain and sweeten with honey and lemon.

Amount to use: 250 ml (1 cup) a day the first week; then increase to 500 ml (2 cups) a day. Drink very slowly.

Rue, Garden Rue

(Ruta graveolins, RUTACEAE.)

Leaves: Blue-green, evergreen lacy, alternate, bi- or tri-pinnate, with leaflets; 1-3 cm (½-1¼ in.) long and 0.5-1 cm (¼-½ in.) wide, crenate, thick and dotted with small immersed oil glands.

Stem: An unusual and beautiful plant, the rue's stem is woody, cylindrical, branched and 0.3-1 m (1-3 ft.) high. Shoots are bluish in spring, turning purplish or brown in winter.

Flowers: Bright yellow or greenish yellow, situated on terminal panicels. Many are 1 cm (½ in.) across. Flowers have 5 petals, curved in at the tips and situated on a disc. The ovary is dotted with glands.

Fruit: Capsule has 4-5 lobes and numerous black seeds.

Taste: Extremely bitter.

Odor: When pinched, the plant emits a disagreeable odor.

Part Used: Leaves, oil.

Habitat: In gardens, wayside areas, pastures, meadows, and sunlit areas of the forest.

Herbal Use

Rue is used to heal rheumatism, arthritis, painful joints, bruises and sprains. Apply the fresh leaves or a compound of oil and dried leaves to the area.

In her book *Elixirs of Life* Mrs. Leyal wrote: "It is said to bestow second sight and it certainly preserves ordinary sight by strengthening the ocular muscles. It acts upon the periosteum and cartilage and removes deposits that through age are liable to form in the tendons and joints, particularly the joints of the wrists. It cures lameness due to sprains, aching tendons, pain in the bones of the feet and ankles."

Do not use during pregnancy.

Tea

How to prepare the tea:

2 ml (½ tsp.) rue
250 ml (1 cup) water

Boil the water and pour it over the herb. Allow to steep for 15 minutes, sweeten with honey, bottle and keep in a cool place.

Amount to use: 125 ml (½ cup) one to two times a day.

Our Fathers of Old

Excellent herbs had our fathers of old —
Excellent herbs to ease their pain —
Alexanders and Marigolds,
Eyebright, Orris, and Elcampane,
Basil, Rosemary, Valerian, Rue,
(Almost singing themselves they run)
Vervain, Dittany, Call-me-to-you
Cowslip, Meliot, Rose of the Sun.

Rudyard Kipling

Sassafras

*(Sassafras officinale; S. varifolium, Laurus Sassafras
LAURACEAE.)*

Leaves: Of varying shape, 10-15 cm (4-6 in.) long, bright green, alternate petiolate, glabrous or smooth on the upper side and downy beneath.

Stem: The plant varies from a shrub in the north to a very tall tree in the south. Stem is generally 3-6 m (10-20 ft.) high and 2-5 cm (1-2 in.) thick and has many slender branches. The wood is light, strong, aromatic and whitish and reddish in colour. The young branches and twigs are smooth and green; the base of the stem and the large branches are greyish, rough, deeply furrowed and divisible into layers.

Flowers: Small greenish yellow racemes that appear before the leaves do; fragrant.

Fruit: Oval, succulent and deep blue; the size of a pea.

Root: Bright orange or brown with a reddish-brown inner surface; irregular curved or quilled pieces; short fracture; with a cork layer and numerous oil cells; about 2-3 cm (1-1¼ in.) thick.

Powder: Reddish brown.

Taste: Sweetish, aromatic.

Odor: Agreeable.

Parts Used: Bark and oil.

Habitat: Grows in temperate and hot climates.

Herbal Use

A stimulant and powerful blood and body cleanser, sassafras is effective in treating rheumatism, sciatica and arthritis; problems of the kidneys, spleen and liver; heart pain; and stomach and intestinal disorders. Sassafras is also used as an after-birth tonic for women.

Tea

Particularly beneficial if you have allergic, tuberculous or rheumatoid arthritis. Do *not* use during pregnancy.

How to prepare the tea:

5 ml (1 tsp.) sassafras bark
250 ml (1 cup) water

Pour water over the herb. Steep 15 minutes, then strain.

Amount to use: 15 ml (1 tbsp.) one to three times a day. Do *not* use for more than two to three weeks.

The stomach is an interesting feature,
That really does exist in every creature,
When it works well you're not aware
That you have any organ there.
But when perchance some food disturbs
'Tis then the time to use my herbs.
Give peppermint for baby's gas,
For older folks use sassafras.
Yes, herbs for me to get me well,
And tell the doctor to go to _____,
No, just say that I don't need him.

93 years oldster

Have Fun With Herbs, by Edith Farwell, p. 96. (Lake Forest, Illinois: Heitman Printing Co., 1958.) Reprinted by permission.

Shiitake Mushrooms

(Lentinus edodes (Berk) Sing; AGARICAE.)

Cap: Light or dark brown with a reddish tinge. The centre is dark and in young specimens the margin is lighter. The cap has a dry surface; large triangular scales; is often fissured, sometimes with large radial fissures; is convex, later depressed around the convex centre; plane in maturity; 4-20 cm (1½-8 in.) broad.

Flesh: White, tough, fleshy in the pileus, hard in the stem.

Lamellae: The gills are a pallid whitish colour, with reddish brown spots appearing in maturity, and have a faint greyish or brownish tinge. They are adnate or adnexed-sinuate but generally soon separate from the stipe, and are crowded close to a thin wavy edge.

Stipe: Light reddish brown, but whitish brown with darker brown scales underneath the attachment of the cortina; solid; thick.

Habitat: Shiitake mushrooms grow on the wood of dead deciduous trees, mainly chestnut, shiia, oak and beech. They fruit all year round where temperature permits. Distributed naturally all over Eastern Asia from China and Japan to Indo-China, shiitake mushrooms do not, however, enter cold or tropical zones. This mushroom is also cultivated in small mushroom farms in British Columbia, the United States, Japan and China.

Herbal Use

Shiitake is one of the finest health-giving plants in the world. Originally it was grown on an evergreen Japanese oak called the "Shii" *(Castanopsis cuspidata)*. For centuries this great mushroom has been commercially cultivated throughout the Orient. It is also one of the great fortunes of the wild mushroom collector. Dr. Kisaku Mori, the world's foremost expert on shiitake mushrooms, writes in his book *Mushrooms as Health Foods* (Tokyo: Japan Publications, Inc.):

The mushroom itself contains proteins, fats, carbohydrates, minerals and vitamins: the spores are especially effective from a medical standpoint. The American specialist Kenneth Cochran has proved that the spores of the shiitake have the ability to create a substance that vigorously resists viruses and that can help cure influenza and cancer.

The enzymes and the bacteria found only in shiitake react in a complex way to produce three kinds of medical effects. They produce a new kind of amino acid that reduces the cholesterol count and lowers blood pressure. Shiitake have the ability to inhibit the growth of viruses and thus to impede their illness-causing activities. Finally, the shiitake contains vitamin B12 and vitamin D2, which are not found in plants and vegetables and which, if eaten by pregnant women, help guarantee strong, healthy newborn babies. In addition, actual cases may be cited in which the shiitake mushroom has been helpful in curing stomach ulcers, duodenal ulcers, leukemia, neuralgia, gout, low blood pressure, amaurosis, myopia, ozena, pyorrhea, constipation and hemorrhoids. It can help recovery from fatigue; in developing greater sexual strength; in promoting general health; and in improving the complexion, the colour of the blood and the appearance of the figure.

The benefits of the fresh mushroom are the same as those of the dried mushroom.

Shiitake mushrooms are an excellent addition to any arthritis healing program.

Tea No. 1

Beneficial for any form of arthritis.

How to prepare the tea:

6 large shiitake mushrooms (fresh)
1 L (1 qt.) water
Dash of soya sauce

Put shiitake mushrooms into water and bring to a boil. Cook for one hour, adding water if necessary. Strain the juice and bottle. Add soya sauce.

Amount to use: Drink 250 ml (1 cup) three to four times a day. May be drunk hot or cold.

Fried Mushrooms

Mushroom stems may be removed and the caps chopped finely. Fry in oil and season with soya sauce. Delicious.

Tansy, Bitter Buttons

(Tanacetum vulgare, COMPOSITAE.)

Leaves: Alternate, dark green, deeply pinnately cleft into narrow and toothed segments, feathery, 15-20 cm (6-8 in.) long and about 10 cm (4 in.) wide. There are up to about 12 segments on each side and one terminal one, attached to a toothed midrib. Segments are smoothish, obtuse, oblong and serrate.

Stem: Straight, leafy, tough, angular, obscurely hexagonal, grooved, 0.3-1 m (1-3 ft.) high and striated. Often reddish in colour.

Flowers: Small, button-like heads of golden yellow flat or tubular florets packed within a depressed involucre. Borne in dense, terminal, flat-topped corymbs. Flowers look as though all the petals have been pulled off, leaving only the central florets.

Fruit: Small and oblong achene with 5-6 ribs and crowned with pappus.

Root: Fibrous, creeping.

Taste: Bitter, pungent.

Odor: Strong, characteristic and disagreeable.

Part Used: Leaves, seeds.

Habitat: Open sunny areas, waysides, pastures and roadways. Tansy is easily identifiable with its carrot-like lacy leaves and bright yellow flowers.

Herbal Use

Tansy is used herbally for rheumatism and arthritis, nervous disorders, kidney and spleen problems, a weak heart, ulcers, tumors, stomach disorders and inflamed eyes. Externally it is also used for joint pain and inflammation.

Do *not* take internally for more than one week at a time. Do not use during pregnancy.

Tea

Excellent for chronic and rheumatoid arthritis.

How to prepare the tea:

5 ml (1 tsp.) tansy leaves
250 ml (1 cup) water

Bring water to a strong boil and pour it over the herb. Allow to stand for 20 minutes. Strain and sweeten with honey. Bottle and store in a cool place.

Amount to use: 125 ml (½ cup) one to three times a day. Do not use for more than one week at a time.

A Garden of Medicinal Flowers

A monk asked Unmon, "What is Dhara Kaya, the formless, timeless, spaceless, ultimate?"

Unmon replied, "A garden of medicinal flowers."

The monk then said, "Is that all I need to understand?"

Unmon replied, "If that isn't enough, then you will have to see the Golden-Haired Lion."

Book of Zen Koans, by Gyomay M. Kubose, p. 56. (Chicago: Contemporary Books, Inc.) Reprinted by permission of the publisher.

White Pond Lily, Sweet Water Lily

(Nymphaea odorate, var. N. alba, var. N. villosa, N. lotus, Nymphaea, NYMPHACEAE.)

Leaves: Up to 25 cm (10 in.) wide, orbicular, floating flat on the water surface, rising from a submerged rhizome. Margin is entire and slightly wavy, with a deep fissure from the margin to the leaf junction making the leaves slightly cordate. The surface is dark green, smooth and shiny. The underside is purple-tinged and has prominent net venation.

Stem: Absent. The flowers grow on long peduncles arising out of the rhizome and the leaves grow on separate petioles up to 6 m (20 ft.) long. All are smooth, tough, flexible and light green and have four equal central canals.

Flowers: Single, large, white or pink-tinged, beautiful and fragrant. The more than 25 petals are elliptical and thick. The petals in the outer row are large; the inner petals are smaller. Flowers are up to 15 cm (6 in.) wide when fully expanded. There are four sepals and a large, fleshy ovary.

Fruit: Globular, fleshy body which retains the stigma and is marked by the scars of petals and stamens which have fallen.

Seeds: 0.2-1.2 cm (less than ½ in.) long, oval, with a sac-like false coat.

Root: Rhizome; thick, tubular, horizontal and elongated, 2.5-7.5 cm (1-3 in.) in diameter and up to 15 cm (6 in.) long. The rhizome is mid to light brown outside and light beige to white inside, with irregular channeling.

Taste: Leaves, spinach-like; rhizome, slightly bitter; seeds, melon-like.

Odor: Sweet and fragrant.

Habitat: Grows in ponds, slow-moving rivers and streams. Blooms from May until October. This aquatic herb grows in all temperate and hot climates of the world. It is widely cultivated in the Orient.

Herbal Use

The white pond lily has been the delight of seers and sages

throughout history. Its mythical, religious and healing qualities have been recorded almost as long as the history of man.

In ancient Egyptian tombs, frescoes depict ceremonies dedicated to the collection and use of this wonderful plant. Special days were allocated for its worship. Many Indian and Asian religions regard it as a sacred symbol for meditation. Deities, especially Buddha, Shili Quan and other bodhisattvas, are often symbolically depicted sitting or standing on a water lily called the Lotus.

In the very early morning, before the sun comes out, the bud of the water lily is closed. As the sun rises, the flower opens.

The water lily is regarded as a staple food in the Orient, where it is widely cultivated. The large, starchy seeds are used in many delicious culinary dishes. The leaves are gathered when young and tender and eaten as a vegetable. The roots, which are rich and starchy, are a favourite vegetable to prepare with chicken. Large roots are usually boiled for a long time to soften their tough fibres. Very young roots have a potato-like quality. The "stalk", which is actually a petiole, is peeled, chopped and boiled like a vegetable.

The seeds, leaves, roots and stalk have different medicinal properties and are prepared in a variety of ways for use in herbal prescriptions.

A blood purifier and tonic to the liver, kidneys and spleen, the white pond lily is effective in treating rheumatism, surface ulcers, pulmonary infections, fevers, skin problems, infected wounds, gall bladder problems, catahrr obstructions and gonorrhea. It is also a diuretic and stimulates inactive bowels.

Tea No. 1

Herbal combination:

30 grams (1 oz.) pond lily root
7 grams (¼ oz.) parsley
15 grams (½ oz.) burdock root

How to prepare the tea:

2 ml (½ tsp.) herb mixture
250 ml (1 cup) water

Pour boiling water over herb. Steep for ½ hour. Strain. Add soya sauce for flavour.

Amount to use: Drink 250 ml (1 cup) one to three times a day.

Tea No. 2

Herbal combination:

30 grams (1 oz.) pond lily root
3 grams (1/10 oz.) cinnamon *(Cinnamonum zeylandicum)*

How to prepare the tea:

2 ml (½ tsp.) herb mixture
250 ml (1 cup) water

Pour boiling water over the herb mixture and allow to steep for ½ hour. Strain and sweeten with honey.

Amount to use: Drink 250 ml (1 cup) one to three times a day.

Tea No. 3

A pain reliever.

Herbal combination:

30 grams (1 oz.) white pond lily root
30 grams (1 oz.) mullein
30 grams (1 oz.) cinnamon *(Cinnamonum zeylandicum)*
30 grams (1 oz.) yarrow *(Achillea millefolium)*

How to prepare the tea: Put the herb mixture into half a litre (1 pint) of water. Simmer for 20 minutes. Strain through a fine cloth.

Amount to use: Drink one small cup (about two tablespoons) twice a day.

Herbal Capsules

Grind the herbs listed in the recipe for Tea. No. 3 into a fine powder. Put into #00 capsules.

Amount to use: Take 3-4 capsules a day.

White Poplar, Quaking Aspen

(Populus tremuloides; SALICACEAE.)

Leaves: 2.5-8 cm (1-3 in.) in diameter, broad, cordate, a lustrous green above and a pale silvery colour below. The leaves quiver in the slightest breeze. In autumn, the leaves turn a brilliant gold or yellow.

Trunk: 6-14 m (6½-15 yds.) high, the trunk is slender—only 0.3-0.6 m (1-2 ft.) in diameter. The tree tapers toward the top and the bark is smooth and coloured greenish-white to cream. On older trees the colour is marked with black warty patches. On young trees the bark is spotted with white and grey or rusty green patches. The internal tissue alternates between buff and white layers. There is a round crown of slender branches.

Buds: Essentially nonresinous.

Taste and Odor: Bitter taste, no odor.

Part Used: Inner bark and leaves.

Habitat: Common in all temperate parts of the world.

Herbal Use

White poplar is used herbally to treat rheumatism and arthritis, swelling of joints, cancer, eczema, colds and bronchial disorders, stomach problems, inflamed eyes, infections and a weak heart. It is also a mild tranquilizer and a liver tonic.

Tea

Herbal combination:

30 grams (1 oz.) white poplar bark
15 grams (½ oz.) golden seal
30 grams (1 oz.) juniper berries
30 grams (1 oz.) uva ursi *(Arctostophylos uva ursi)*
30 grams (1 oz.) comfrey
15 grams (½ oz.) ginger
30 grams (1 oz.) mullein

How to prepare the tea:

15 ml (3 tsp.) herb mixture
1 L (1 qt.) water

Put all herbs into a mortar and grind to a fine powder. Put the herbs into the boiling water and allow to steep for three hours. Strain through a fine cloth. Use yogurt in the diet the same day. Store in a cool place.

Amount to use: 125 ml (½ cup) one to three times a day.

Maitri Upanishad VI, 13

Now this, too, has been said elsewhere: The form of the Lord Vishnu known as "supporter of all" is nothing less than food. The breath of life is the sap *(rassa)* of food; mind of life; the understanding *(vijnana)* of mind; bliss, of the understanding. The man who knows this will come to possess food, the breath of life, mind, understanding and bliss; knowing this, he will eat the food of as many beings as eat food here on earth, for he will indwell them:

Food overcomes decay,
It is full of charm they say:
Food is the breath of life in beasts;
Food is the foremost, food the healer:
Such is the tradition handed down.

Hindu Scriptures, p. 231. (Toronto, Ontario: J.M. Dent and Sons (Canada) Ltd.) Reprinted by permission of the publisher.

Wild Ginseng, Sarsaparilla

(Aralia nudicaulis; ARALIACEAE.)

This herb is similar to the Oriental ginseng described earlier, with the following exceptions. The seeds and berries of the wild plant appear before the leaves do in the early spring. The leaf is also more elongated and the root is longer and slimmer in the wild plant.

This herb grows abundantly in parts of British Columbia and is used by the Northwest Coast Indians for stomach complaints. The Hopi in California have regarded this plant as sacred for the last two centuries and hold regular spring ceremonies for the gathering and preserving of this precious herb.

Wild ginseng can be found on the north side of mountains at elevations over 3,000 feet.

Herbal Use

Wild ginseng is used in the same manner as the cultivated ginseng described earlier. It will act beneficially in any arthritis or rheumatism healing program.

PART THREE:
ORIENTAL ORIGINS
OF HERBAL HEALING

Prevention: An Ancient Tradition

The art of herbal healing was developed in the ancient Far East. For the past two thousand years of the Orient's rich medical tradition (which spans, in all, more than 4,500 years), Oriental doctors have emphasized preventive medicine. Rather than waiting for symptoms to appear and then seeking a cure, they believed that a person should include in his or her daily diet certain foods which would prevent illness. In the words of the great herbalist Chang-Chung Ching: "Forestalling the illness and treating it before it is apparent is the work of a superior order." Oriental philosophy makes no distinction between food and medicine. Herbs used to season and enhance food are, like food, medicine.

Although one need not know Chinese philosophy or tradition to benefit from the medical knowledge it has given us, it is nevertheless helpful to understand something of the context within which Chinese herbalists developed their art.

Oriental Philosophy of Medicine

The early Chinese doctors belonged to the royal courts or the monastic orders, where they maintained the tradition of making medicines and recorded their prescriptions. Philosophical works such as the *I Ching* (Book of Changes), the *Shu Ching* and the *Tao* exerted great influence on their thinking, providing the framework through which they saw man and the universe.

The *I Ching*, one of the world's oldest books (early fragments have been dated at 1000 B.C.), introduced a basic concept in Oriental thought—the interplay of Yin and Yang. Yin and Yang are the two opposing elements in the world from which all phenomena are created by their constant interplay. Yin is negative, dark, cold and feminine; Yang is positive, light, warm and masculine.

When a person is in good health, his body is in a condition of equilibrium. Any imbalance affects the whole organism—if the body is too Yang it becomes overpowerful, with increased activity and overexertion. If the body is too Yin, the result is hypofunction and withdrawal.

Although the earliest comprehensive medical books were written by the Chinese two thousand years ago, most did not reach the outside world until the 1500s, when Portuguese and English explorers and traders began the exchange of goods and ideas between Europe and the Middle Kingdom. From that time until the eighteenth century, many European medical prescriptions were based on Oriental traditions.

Many of the great Western medical discoveries after the 1850s—anesthesia, penicillin, and smallpox vaccination, for example—had their Oriental counterparts as early as the second century and probably earlier. Circulation of the blood, not known in Europe until the late 1500s, was described in the *Yellow Emperors Classic*, written about A.D. 100. As early as the sixth century B.C., Oriental doctors were taking their patients' pulses. In many instances ancient Oriental doctors were treating diseases with specific remedies which have only in the past decade been confirmed by modern science.

But most ancient practitioners were not primarily interested in analysis or research. They devoted their energies to making prescriptions, some of which took years to prepare, and were more concerned with maintaining existing knowledge than with discovering new healing processes. A poem from the court of Prince Huai Nan, A.D. 1, sums up this attitude.

> The sun and moon move around
> their courses, time waits for nobody.
> Therefore the sage values a whole
> foot of jade less than one inch
> of sun shadow. Time is easily lost
> and hard to get.
>
> *Chia*

Early Oriental Medicine Books

By the end of the Shang Dynasty (1766-1123 B.C.), the Chinese and Japanese were very knowledgeable about herbal therapy and had compiled numerous classics. Books as old as 2,000 years were in existence.

The *Book of Ode,* one of the early literary Chinese works, recorded plant herbs many of which are still in use today.

Another ancient book, *Classic of Mountain and Ocean,* introduced mineral drugs and drugs of animal origin as well as those from plants. It recorded over a hundred herbs and the treatment for many diseases.

Shennongs Materia Medica, the most famous classic of the Han Dynasty (206 B.C.-A.D. 221), described 365 herbs of plant, animal and mineral origin. Each was categorized according to its actions. The book also listed 170 diseases treated by herbs. This classic and Li Shi-chen's medical books (see below) laid the groundwork of Oriental herbal therapy and are still considered accurate in the treatment of disease today.

The *Yellow Emperors Classic of Internal Medicine,* mentioned earlier, was written about A.D. 100. It is especially noteworthy for its description of the circulation of the blood.

The first book to reach the West was the *Pen-ts'ao Kang-mu,* compiled about 1578 by the doctor and pharmacist Li Shi-chen. A study of all the medical research in China up to that time, it described 1,892 different medicaments and 10,000 medical prescriptions. This comprehensive work was translated into Japanese, Latin, French, Russian, English, German and other languages.

The next important book, published in 1590 and also written by Li Shi-chen, was *Ch'i-chung Pa-mai,* or *Eight Special Meridians.* This was the first book to describe the part played by the pulse and the special meridians and lines in the body. These meridians were later established to be the same as those used in acupuncture. The collection of Li Shi-chen's works is titled *An Outline of Materia Medica.*

The *I-tsung Chin-chien,* or *The Golden Mirror of the Art of Healing,* was first published in 1749. It was a collection of the works of eighty leading doctors and the most important of the hundreds of works produced during the Ch'ing period.

In the 1600s *Materia Medica* was taken to Japan. A few years later it was translated into Japanese by a great Japanese physician named Onono. The twenty volumes, published in 1783, subsequently formed the basis for Japanese herbology. Updated and translated again in 1929, it is still a major reference work to many Japanese physicians today.

Man and the Universe

Chinese herbalists, like the philosophers, saw man as an integral and organic part of the universe. They believed that the same laws applied to both man and nature; man was the microcosm directly affected by nature, the macrocosm. The early concept of process, which the Chinese attributed to the human organism with all its ills, was the interrelationship and interplay of the five basic elements: fire, earth, metal, water and wood. These elements could work against each other in a destructive way, or they could work together in a mutually beneficial relationship.

Creative cycle

Fire creates earth
Earth creates metal
Metal creates water
Water creates wood
Wood creates fire

Destructive cycle

Wood destroys earth   (by covering it)
Fire destroys metal   (by melting it)
Earth destroys water   (by retaining it)
Metal destroys wood   (by cutting it)
Water destroys fire   (by extinguishing it)

Chi energy is another important Oriental concept. Said Su Wen, a philosopher and herbalist: "Essential primordial energy gives birth to all the elements and is integrated into them." This the Orientals called Chi energy.

After centuries of observation, it was noted that Chi energy is present in the body and always follows a certain course. Throughout the day, each organ in the body experiences two hours of Yin (or weak) energy and two hours of Yang (or powerful) energy.

Chi energy is used today to locate imbalances in the body and acupuncture points.

Herbal Healing

Because man is part of the natural universe, the food he eats has either a Yin or Yang effect on his body.

Although modern medical chemicals help in many cases to cure disease, they do not possess the same healing qualities found in herbal prescriptions. A plant, piece of bark, or berry may contain up to twenty ingredients which interact to produce a healing effect. Most modern drugs consist of one or more isolated molecules surrounded by a sugar base. This type of medicine often leaves the body in a very Yin condition—the body must expend greater energy to utilize the chemical because it is not aided by the ingredients which naturally interact with the chemical.

In most instances, it takes longer to remove a disease using the ancient methods than it does to use modern drugs. But herbal healing has few side effects or complications, its benefits are longer lasting and it usually leaves the body in a healthier condition. Herbal regimens aim to maintain the body's overall health while healing is taking place.

Traditional Oriental healers consider modern doctors authorities to consult in an emergency or, as they call them, "accident doctors." Their own healing processes take an entirely different approach, emphasizing lifelong dietary habits. Herbalists have never claimed that any one herb cures any one disease. What herbs do is to stimulate the resistance of the body's own tissue to the disease or condition. Health and disease cannot dominate the body at the same time.

Glossary

Achene: One-seeded fruit, dry, small; remains closed at maturity.

Acute: In a leaf, terminating in a sharp point.

Adnate: One part of a plant that is different, but attached to the same plant, *e.g.* bracts attached to the receptacle.

Alternate: Not opposite; attached singly along the stem.

Annual: Living for only one growing season.

Annulate: Has rings formed by each year's growth.

Anther: Top part of the stamen that produces and bears the pollen.

Apex: The tip of a leaf or plant.

Axil: The upper angle formed by a branch or leaf with the stem.

Axillary: Situated in the axil of a leaf or bract.

Basal: Located at the base of the stem.

Berry: A single ovary; fleshy fruit.

Biennial: Living for only two growing seasons. Fruit and flowers are usually produced in the second year.

Blade: The expanded, flat part of a leaf.

Bract: A very small or modified leaf, usually growing at the base of a leaf or flower cluster.

Bud: An unexpanded flower or leaf.

Bulb: An underground leaf bud with fleshy scales.

Calyx: A term used to describe the sepals collectively; the outer green whorl at the outside of a flower petal.

Cambium: The layer of cells between the bark and the wood.

Campanulate: Shaped like a bell.

Capsule: A dry fruit, opening at maturity into two or more sections.

Catkin: An elongated petalless flower, usually drooping.

Cell: A very small complex vestical from which living organisms are formed.

Cleft: Deeply incised or cut.

Compound: Has two or more similar parts.

Compound leaf: Where two or more similar leaves have a common stalk.

Cordate: Heart-shaped.

Corolla: The part of a flower made up of petals, either individual or joined together.

Cortex: The outer bark or skin.

Corymb: A flat-topped flower cluster in which the outer flower opens first.

Crenate: Even or uneven dentate with round teeth.

Crown: The leafy top of a tree or plant.

Cyme: A flat-topped, branched flower. The middle flowers open first.

Cymose: Having cymes, or cyme-like.

Deciduous: A plant or tree which loses its leaves every year.

Dentate: With teeth along the edge.

Decurrent: When the gills of a mushroom or plant are prolonged down the stem.

Decussate: Alternating at right angles in pairs at the different levels.

Depressed: Slightly hollowed.

Elliptical: Having the form of an ellipse.

Entire: A leaf margin which is even and untoothed.

Epidermal: The surface layer of cells.

Fibrous: Composed of fibres; composed of elongated thick-celled walls.

Filament: The long and slender part of a stamen.

Fissure: Split in the surface.

Floret: A very small flower, usually part of a flower, *e.g.* dandelion.

Fractures: Breaks or splits on the surface of the wood; irregular with a fractured appearance.

Fruit: The seed-bearing body of a plant; ovary of a plant.

Fusiform: Shaped like a spindle, swollen in the middle and tapering toward the ends.

Glabrous: Smooth.

Globose: Round, like a globe.

Granular: Has minute grains.

Head: A group of florets or flowers joined together in a short dense terminal cluster, *e.g.* clover.

Imbricate: Overlapping so that the lower piece covers the base of the next higher piece.

Inflorescence: A group of flowers.

Involucre: The circle of bracts surrounding or beneath a flower cluster or a single flower.

Lanceolate: Shaped like a lance; long leaves that taper at the apex.

Leaflet: One of the separate but similar parts of a divided leaf.

Legume: Fruit of the *LEGUMINOSAE*, produced from a unilocular ovary.

Margin: Pertaining to the edge of a leaf or mushroom.

Net veined: Veins on a leaf are close and net-like.

Oblong: Longer than wide, with parallel sides.

Obovate: Inversely ovate.

Obtuse: Blunt or rounded at the end.

Opposite: Growing directly across from each other at the same node.

Oval: Broadly elliptical; broader near the middle and rounded at both ends.

Ovary: The enlarged part of the pistil that produces the seeds.

Ovate: Flat and egg-shaped with the widest part near the base.

Ovoid: A solid with an ovate outline.

Palmate: Veins or lobes radiating out from a common point.

Palmately compound: A compound leaf with the leaflets arising from the same point, *e.g.* horse chestnut.

Palmately lobed: Cleft or divided to give the leaf a palmate configuration.

Panicle: An elongated flower cluster.

Papilionaceous: Butterfly-like flowers with wings, *e.g.* the pea family.

Pappus: Bristles or hairs on top of the fruit of the *COMPOSITAE* family.

Pedicel: The stalk of a single flower.

Peduncle: The flower stalk supporting a cluster or solitary flower.

Perennial: A plant which lives more than two years.

Perianth: The calyx and corolla surrounding the stamens and pistil.

Petal: One or more segments of the corolla.

Petiole: The stem or stalk of a leaf.

Pileus: The cap of a mushroom.

Pinnate: Compound, with the leaflets arranged on each side of a common axis.

Pinnately compound: Cleft or divided, so as to give the leaf a feather-like configuration.

Pistil: Part of a flower containing the ovary.

Pith: The central softer part of a twig or leaf stalk.

Plane: With a flat surface.

Pod: A dry fruit, as those of the pea family.

Quilled: Applied to florets which have become tubular.

Raceme: An elongated flower cluster with stalked flowers arranged along a central stem.

Radial: Diverging from a central point.

Radiate: Spreading outward from a common centre.

Receptacle: The enlarged or expanded end of a stem to which the parts of a flower are attached.

Reticulate: In the form of a network; net veined.

Rhizome: An underground stem, often fleshy, *e.g.* ginger.

Rib: A primary or prominent vein of a leaf.

Rosette: A cluster of radiating leaves or other part of a plant.

Runcinate: Sharply incised, with the segments directed backward.

Scale: Any thin body, sometimes of epidermal origin.

Sepal: Floral bract, green and leaf-like.

Serrate: Saw-toothed, pointing outwards.

Sessile: Attached directly to the base, without a stalk.

Simple: Not compound.

Sinuate: With the margin very wavy.

Spike: A simple inflorescence of stalkless flowers arranged along a central stem.

Stamen: The male organ of a flower consisting of a slender stalk and a pollen-bearing anther.

Stigma: The top of a pistil.

Stipe: The stem supporting the cap of a fungus.

Stipule: A small leaf-like growth, usually in pairs, at the base of a leaf stalk.

Stomata: A minute orifice or mouth-like opening between the two guard cells in the epidermis, usually on the lower surface of the leaf.

Striate: Marked with fine longitudinal lines.

Strobile: An inflorescence, marked by imbricated bracts or scales, *e.g.* hops.

Style: The stalk of a pistil.

Subglobular: Somewhat rounded.

Terminal: At the end or apex of a stem or branch.

Trailing: Running along the ground but not rooting.

Trifoliate: Having three leaflets.

Umbel: A flower cluster in which all the flower stalks radiate from the same point.

Undulate: Wavy surface or margin.

Vein: One of a network of tiny channels in a leaf through which the plant fluids flow.

Venation: The character of veining.

Whorled: Arranged in a circle around a central point.

Roots

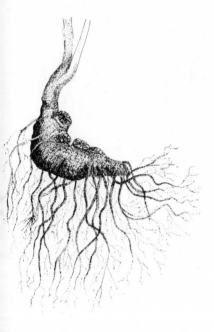

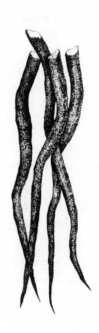

Black Cohosh

Burdock

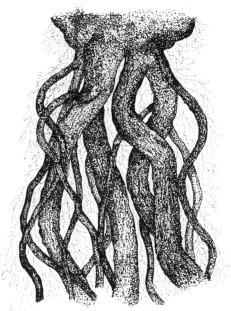

Comfrey

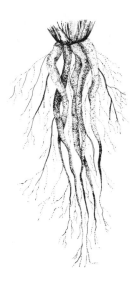

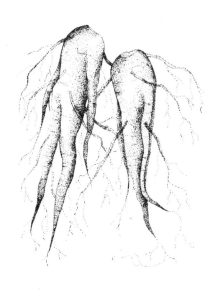

Dandelion   Ginseng

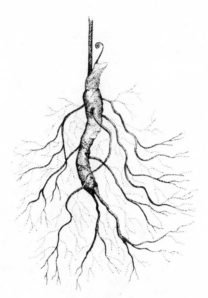

Golden Seal

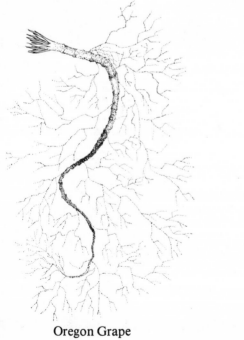

Oregon Grape

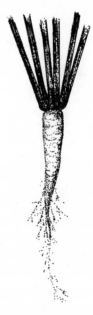

Parsley

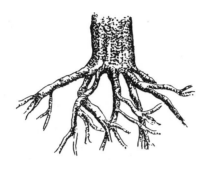

Woody root

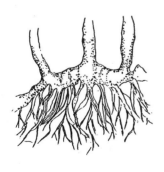

Perennial root

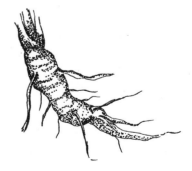

Fleshy root

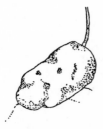

Root tuber

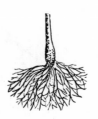

Fibrous root

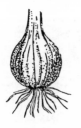

Bulb

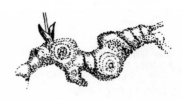

Rhizome

Leaves

Form

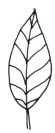 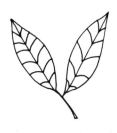

Simple   Compound

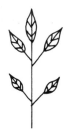 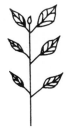

Odd pinnately
compound

Even pinnately
compound

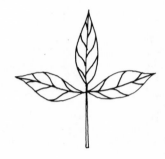

Trifoliate compound

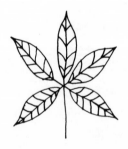

Palmately compound

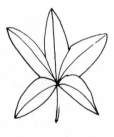

Palmately cleft

Margin

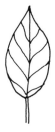

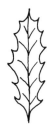

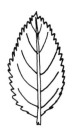

Entire   Dentate   Serrate

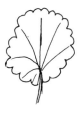

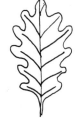

Crenate   Undulate

Shape

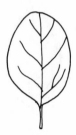

Oval

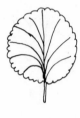

Round

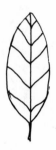

Ovate

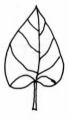

Cordate

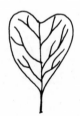

Obcordate

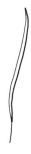 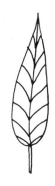 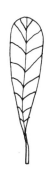

Needle   Lanceolate   Oblanceolate

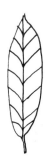 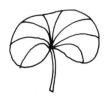

Oblong   Reinform

Venation

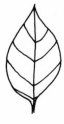
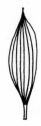
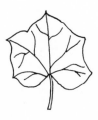

Pinnate   Parallel   Radiate

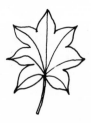
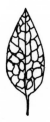

Palmate   Net

Inflorescences

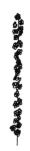
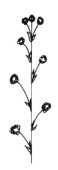
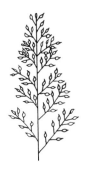

Spike   Panicle   Corymb

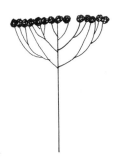
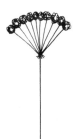
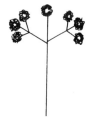

Umbel   Racemose   Cymose

Flower

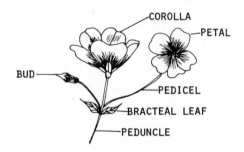

COROLLA

PETAL

BUD

PEDICEL

BRACTEAL LEAF

PEDUNCLE

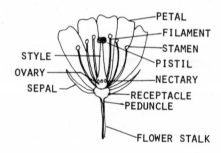

PETAL

FILAMENT

STAMEN

STYLE

PISTIL

OVARY

NECTARY

SEPAL

RECEPTACLE

PEDUNCLE

FLOWER STALK

Bibliography

Aichele, Dietmar. *Wild Flowers.* London W.1: Octopus Books, 1973.

Beatie, Piper. *The Flora of the Northwest Coast.* Lancaster, Pa.: New Era Printing Company, 1915.

Brockman, C.F. *Trees of North America.* New York, N.Y.: Golden Press, 1968.

Chen, Prof. C.Y. *History of Chinese Medical Science.* Hong Kong: Hong Kong Press, 1967.

Christopher, Dr. John. *School of Natural Healing.* Provo, Utah: Microlith Printing, 1976.

Chung-Yuan, Chang. *Original Teachings of Chan Buddhism.* Toronto: Vintage Books Edition, Random House of Canada Limited, 1971.

Coon, Nelson. *Using Plants for Healing.* New York: Hearthside Press Inc., 1963.

Dash, Bhagwan. *Tibetan Medicine.* Dharamsala, Himachal Pradesh, India: Library of Tibetan Works and Archives, 1976.

Ehret, Arnold. *Mucusless Diet Healing System.* California: Ehret Literature Publishing Company, Beaumont Publishing, 1922.

Elliot, Douglas B. *Roots.* Old Greenwich, Conn.: Chatham Press, 1976.

Enari, Leonid. *Plants of the Pacific Northwest.* Portland, Oregon: Binfords and Mort Publishers, 1956.

Fluck, Hans. *Medicinal Plants and Their Uses.* Yeovil Road, Slough, Berks, England: W. Foulsham and Co. Ltd., 1973.

Fritz, Martin Engel. *Flora Magica.* Munchen, Germany: Keysersche, Verlagsbuchhandlung, 1966.

Gleason, Henry A. *New Britton & Brow Illustrated Flora,* Vol. 3. Lancaster, Pa.: Lancaster Press Inc., 1952.

Goodale, George L., M.D. *Wild Flowers of America.* Bradlee Whidden, 1886.

Greive, Mrs. M. *A Modern Herbal.* London, England: Jonathan Cape, 30 Bedford Square, 1931.

Han, Shi Sheng. *Chi Min Yao Sui.* (Trans.) 6th century. Peking, China: Science Press, 1962.

Harrington, H.D. *Edible Native Plants of the Rocky Mountains.* The University of New Mexico Press, 1967.

Haskin, Leslie L. *Wild Flowers of the Pacific Coast.* Portland, Oregon: Binfords and Mort, Publishers, 1967.

Health, Medicine Co. *The Principles and Practical Use of Acupuncture Anaesthesia.* Hong Kong: Medicine and Health Publishing Co., 1974.

Hsu, Hong-Yen. *The Studies of Chinese Herb Medicine.* Republic of China: Chinese Herb Medicine Committee, 1972.

Hudson, Irene Bastow. *Medicinal and Food Plants of British Columbia.* Victoria, B.C.: Quality Press Printers, 1950.

Hutchens, Alma. *Indian Herbology of North America.* Windsor, Ontario: Merco, 620 Wyandotte E., 1974.

Hylander, Clarence J. *Wild Flower Book.* New York, N.Y.: The MacMillan Co., 1954.

Jain, S.K. *Medicinal Plants.* New Delhi, India: National Books Trust, 1968.

Jensen, Bernard. *The Herbalist.* Provo, Utah: Bi-World publishers, P.O. Box 62.

Johnson, Lawrence. *Medical Botany of North America.* New York: William Wood and Co.; London: 56 and 58 Lafayette Place, 1884.

Kelsang, Jhampa. *The Ambrosia Heart Tantra.* Dharamsala, Himachal Pradesh, India: Library of Tibetan Works and Archives, 1977.

Kirk, Donald. *Wild Edible Plants of the Western United States.* Healdsburg, Calif.: Naturegraph Publishers, 1970.

Kulvinskas, Viktoras. *Survival into the 21st Century.* Wethersfield, Conn.: Omagod Press, P.O. Box 255, 1977.

Law, Donald. *Herbs for Cooking and for Healing.* London: W. Foulsham and Co. Ltd., 1970.

Le Maout, E. *Botany.* London: Longmans, Green and Co., 1876.

Lewis, Walter H. *Medical Botany.* New York; Toronto, Ontario: John Wiley and Sons Ltd., 1977.

Liu, Da. *Tai Chi Ch'uan and I Ching.* New York: Harper and Row Publishing Co., 10 E. 53rd St.

Liu, Da. *Taoist Health Exercise Book.* New York, N.Y.: Links Press, 1974.

Lu, Henry. *Introduction to Chinese Classics in Medicine.* Vancouver, B.C.: Academy of Oriental Heritage, P.O. Box 35057, Station E.

Lucas, Richard. *Nature's Medicines.* New York, N.Y.: Park Publishing Co. Inc., 1966.

Lucas, Richard. *Secrets of the Chinese Herbalists.* West Nyack, N.Y.: Parker Publishing Inc., 1977.

Lyons, C.P. *Trees, Shrubs and Flowers to know in British Columbia.* Bath, England: Sir Isaac Pitman and Son, Pitman Press, 1956.

Mori, Kisaku. *Mushrooms as Health Foods.* San Francisco, Ca.: Japan Publications Trading Co., 1974.

Mary, Jean. *L'Armoire aux Herbes.* Paris, France: Loes Ecrits de France, 22 Rue Bergere, 1966.

Medsger, Oliver Perry. *Edible Wild Plants.* New York, N.Y.: The MacMillan Co., 1944.

Millspaugh, Charles F. *American Medicinal Plants.* New York, N.Y.: Dover Publications Inc., 1892.

Muenscher, Walter Conrad. *Poisonous Plants of the United States.* New York, N.Y.: The MacMillan Co., 1939.

Numata, Makoto. *Biological Flora of Japan.* Tokyo, Japan: Tsuki Shokan Publishing Co., 2-82 Tsuki Chuo-Ku, 1972.

Ogura, Ryozo. *Zen Koans.* Chicago, Illinois: Henry Regnery Co., 1973.

Palmer, E. *Fieldbook of Natural History.* New York: McGraw Hill, 1975.

Pen, Tsao Kang Mu. *Chinese Medical Journal,* Vol. 6: 174-191, 1956.

Prabhavananda, Swami. *The Upanishads.* Hollywood, Calif.: Vedanta Press, 1946 Vendanta Place, 1948.

Rendel, Alfred Barton. *The Classification of Flowering Plants.* London: Cambridge University Press, 1952.

Riolle, Trouard. *Les Plantes Medicinales.* Paris, France: Flammarion, 26 Rue Racine, 1964.

Romance of Empire Drugs, The. London, England: Stafford Allen and Sons Ltd., Cowper Street, 1953.

Singer, Rolf. *Mushrooms and Truffles.* London, England: Leonard Hill Books Ltd., 1961.

Smith, Dr. F. Porter. *Chinese Medica.* Tai Pei, Taiwan: Kun T'ing Book House, 1969.

Stewart, Harold. *A Chime of Windbells.* (Trans.) Tokyo, Japan: Charles E. Tuttle Co., Publishers, 1965.

Tampon, John. *Dangerous Plants.* New York, N.Y.: Universe Books, 1977.

Tobe, John H. *The Miracle of Live Juices and Raw Foods.* St. Catherines, Ontario: Provoker Press, 1976.

Turner, Nancy. *Food Plants of B.C. Indians.* Victoria: British Columbia Provincial Museum, 1975.

Turner, Szczawinski. *Edible Garden Weeds of Canada.* Ottawa: National Museums of Natural Sciences, 1978.

Veninga and Zaricor. *Golden Seal.* Santa Cruz, Ca.: Ruka Publications, P.O. Box 1072, 1978.

Waley, Arthur. *The Nine Songs.* San Francisco, California: City Lights Books, 1955.

Watt, John Mitchell. *The Medicinal and Poisonous Plants of Southern and Eastern Africa.* Edinburgh and London: E. & S. Livingstone Ltd., 1962.

Willfort, Richard. *Gesundheit Durch Heilkrauter.* Linz, Austria: Rudolf Trauner Verlag, 1967.

Williams, Trevor Illtyd. *Drugs from Plants.* London, England: A.S. Atkinson Ltd., 154 Clerkenwell Road, 1947.

Wren, R.C. *Potters New Encyclopedia of Medicinal Herbs.* New York, N.Y.: Harper & Row, 1972.

Youngken, Herbert W. *Pharmaceutical Botany.* Toronto, Ontario: The Blackstone Company, 1951.

Zachner, R.C. *Hindu Scriptures.* (Trans.) New York: J.M. Dent and Sons, Ltd., 1966.

Index

Ailments and Symptoms

Herbs